Sexual Health, Fertility, and Relationships in Cancer Care

PSYCHO-ONCOLOGY CARE SERIES: COMPANION GUIDES FOR CLINICIANS

Series Co-Editors: David W. Kissane and Maggie Watson

Published and Forthcoming Titles:

Management of Clinical Depression and Anxiety

Sexual Health, Fertility, and Relationships in Cancer Care

Psycho-Oncology in Palliative and End-of-Life Care

Cancer Survivorship and Health Promotion

Sexual Health, Fertility, and Relationships in Cancer Care

Edited by
Maggie Watson, PhD
Honorary Research Associate
Section of Onco-Genetics, Institute of Cancer Research
Sutton and London, UK
Honorary Professor
Research Department of Clinical, Educational and Health Psychology
University College London
London, UK
and
David W. Kissane, AC, MD, FRANZCP, FAChPM, FACLP
Professor of Psychiatry
University of Notre Dame, Australia
Chair of Palliative Medicine Research
Cunningham Centre, St. Vincent's Hospital
Sydney, Australia
Head of Szalmuk Family Psycho-Oncology Research Unit
Cabrini Health
Emeritus Professor of Psychiatry
Monash University
Melbourne, Australia

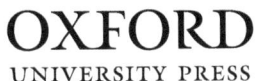

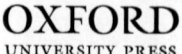

UNIVERSITY PRESS

Oxford University Press is a department of the University of Oxford. It furthers
the University's objective of excellence in research, scholarship, and education
by publishing worldwide. Oxford is a registered trade mark of Oxford University
Press in the UK and certain other countries.

Published in the United States of America by Oxford University Press
198 Madison Avenue, New York, NY 10016, United States of America.

© Oxford University Press 2020

All rights reserved. No part of this publication may be reproduced, stored in
a retrieval system, or transmitted, in any form or by any means, without the
prior permission in writing of Oxford University Press, or as expressly permitted
by law, by license, or under terms agreed with the appropriate reproduction
rights organization. Inquiries concerning reproduction outside the scope of the
above should be sent to the Rights Department, Oxford University Press, at the
address above.

You must not circulate this work in any other form
and you must impose this same condition on any acquirer.

Library of Congress Cataloging-in-Publication Data
Names: Watson, Maggie, editor. | Kissane, David W. (David William), editor.
Title: Sexual health, fertility, and relationships in Cancer Care /
[edited by] Maggie Watson and David W. Kissane.
Other titles: Psycho-oncology care.
Description: New York, NY : Oxford University Press, [2020] |
Series: Psycho-oncology care: companion guides for clinicians |
Includes bibliographical references and index.
Identifiers: LCCN 2019054247 (print) | LCCN 2019054248 (ebook) |
ISBN 9780190934033 (paperback) | ISBN 9780190934057 (epub) |
ISBN 9780190934064 (online)
Subjects: MESH: Sexual Health | Psycho-Oncology—methods | Sexual
Dysfunctions, Psychological—therapy | Fertility | Interpersonal Relations
Classification: LCC RA788 (print) | LCC RA788 (ebook) | NLM WM 620 |
DDC 613.9/5—dc23
LC record available at https://lccn.loc.gov/2019054247
LC ebook record available at https://lccn.loc.gov/2019054248

This material is not intended to be, and should not be considered, a substitute for
medical or other professional advice. Treatment for the conditions described in this
material is highly dependent on the individual circumstances. And, while this material
is designed to offer accurate information with respect to the subject matter covered
and to be current as of the time it was written, research and knowledge about medical
and health issues is constantly evolving and dose schedules for medications are being
revised continually, with new side effects recognized and accounted for regularly.
Readers must therefore always check the product information and clinical procedures
with the most up-to-date published product information and data sheets provided by
the manufacturers and the most recent codes of conduct and safety regulation. The
publisher and the authors make no representations or warranties to readers, express
or implied, as to the accuracy or completeness of this material. Without limiting the
foregoing, the publisher and the authors make no representations or warranties as to
the accuracy or efficacy of the drug dosages mentioned in the material. The authors
and the publisher do not accept, and expressly disclaim, any responsibility for any
liability, loss, or risk that may be claimed or incurred as a consequence of the use
and/or application of any of the contents of this material

Preface

Psycho-oncology is a sub-specialty of oncology which focuses on psychosocial problems experienced by cancer patients and their families and carers; it provides evidence-based approaches to management of these specific problems.

These *Companion Guides in Psycho-Oncology Care* are intended to make clinical management information accessible to either oncology clinical staff, who may not have had specialized mental health training, or those professionals still in training as mental health specialists seeking to increase their psycho-oncology skills.

Mental health problems in cancer patients can be both pre-existing and arise within the context of the cancer's diagnosis and treatment. This companion guide covers sexual health, fertility, and relationships in cancer care and provides information relating to diagnosis, treatment, and service issues presented in a brief condensed format, which can be used as a quick access source to support clinical decision-making. Sexuality and fertility can be major challenges for many couples and vital information to guide diagnosis and management is presented here.

The authors of this *Companion Guide* are experienced clinicians and researchers with many years of experience in the care of patients with cancer and their families. We thank them for sharing this expertise. As editors, we also thank the staff of Oxford University Press for their support and the International Psycho-Oncology Society for their assistance with distribution.

The psychosocial care of cancer patients and their families is a basic human right. We hope that the readers of this book will find it helpful to advance the quality of this care delivery to thus enrich the lives of all patients with cancer and their families.

Maggie Watson, PhD
David W. Kissane, MD

Contents

Contributors *ix*

1. **Provision of Onco-Fertility Support** *1*
   Roxana Schwab, Andrea Kiemen, Joachim Weis, and Annette Hasenburg

2. **Provision of Sexual Health Support** *19*
   Jane M. Ussher, Alexandra Hawkey, and Janette Perz

3. **Lesbian, Gay, Bisexual, and Transgender Issues** *41*
   Karolina Lisy, Nick Hulbert-Williams, Jane M. Ussher, Alison Alpert, Charles Kamen, and Michael Jefford

4. **Adolescents and Young Adults** *63*
   Catherine Benedict, Zeba Ahmad, Vicky Lehmann, and Jennifer S. Ford

5. **Principles of Treatment of Sexual Dysfunction** *98*
   Michelle Peate and Ilona Juraskova

6. **Psychological Treatment of Individual Sexual Dysfunction** *115*
   Daniela Wittmann

7. **Couple Therapy for Sexual Dysfunction** *139*
   Talia I. Zaider and David W. Kissane

Index *159*

Contributors

Zeba Ahmad
Health Psychology & Clinical Science
Hunter College and the Graduate
  Center
City University of New York
New York, NY

Alison Alpert
University of Rochester
  Medical Centre
Rochester, New York, NY

Catherine Benedict
Clinical Assistant Professor
Psychiatry & Behavioral Sciences
Stanford School of Medicine
Palo Alto, CA

Jennifer S. Ford
Professor
Department of Psychology
Hunter College and the Graduate
  Center
City University of New York
New York, NY

Annette Hasenburg
Head of Department, Head of
  Oncology Centre
Mainz University Medical Center
Mainz, Germany

Alexandra Hawkey
Translational Health Research
  Institute, School of Medicine
Western Sydney University, Australia

Nick Hulbert-Williams
Professor of Behavioural Medicine
Centre for Contextual Behavioural
  Science, School of Psychology
University of Chester
Chester, Cheshire, UK

Michael Jefford
Consultant Medical Oncologist
Department of Medical Oncology
Peter MacCallum Cancer Centre
Melbourne, VIC, Australia

Ilona Juraskova
Associate Professor in Health
  Psychology
Psychology
The University of Sydney
Sydney, NSW, Australia

Charles Kamen
University of Rochester
  Medical Centre
Rochester, New York, NY

Andrea Kiemen
Senior Researcher
Interdisciplinary Tumor
  Center–Comprehensive
  Cancer Centre
Endowed Professorship for
  Self-help Research
Freiburg, Baden-Württemberg,
  Germany

**David W. Kissane, AC, MD,
FRANZCP, FAChPM, FACLP**
Professor of Psychiatry
University of Notre Dame, Australia
Chair of Palliative Medicine Research
Cunningham Centre, St. Vincent's
  Hospital
Sydney, Australia
Head of Szalmuk Family Psycho-
  Oncology Research Unit
Cabrini Health
Emeritus Professor of Psychiatry
Monash University
Melbourne, Australia

Vicky Lehmann
Senior Researcher
Department of Medical Psychology
Amsterdam University Medical Centers, University of Amsterdam
Amsterdam, The Netherlands

Karolina Lisy
Australian Cancer Survivorship Centre
Peter MacCallum Cancer Centre
Melbourne, VIC, Australia

Michelle Peate
Program Leader, Psychosocial Health and Wellbeing Research (emPoWeR) Unit
Department of Obstetrics and Gynaecology
University of Melbourne
Parkville, VIC, Australia

Janette Perz
Translational Health Research Institute, School of Medicine
Western Sydney University
Sydney, NSW, Australia

Roxana Schwab
Head of Gynecologic Dysplasia Unit
Mainz University Medical Center
Mainz, Germany

Jane M. Ussher
Translational Health Research Institute, School of Medicine
Western Sydney University
Sydney, NSW, Australia

Joachim Weis
Professor, Peer-Support Research
Medical Faculty and University Clinic Freiburg Comprehensive Cancer Center
Freiburg, Germany

Daniela Wittmann
Associate Professor
Department of Urology
Adjunct Associate Professor
School of Social Work
University of Michigan
Ann Arbor, MI

Talia I. Zaider
Assistant Attending Psychologist and Director
Family Therapy Clinic
Department of Psychiatry & Behavioral Sciences
Memorial Sloan Kettering Cancer Center
New York, NY

Chapter 1

Provision of Onco-Fertility Support

Roxana Schwab, Andrea Kiemen, Joachim Weis, and Annette Hasenburg

Learning Objectives

After reading this chapter the clinician will be able to:

1. Realize that onco-fertility care is a complex and challenging task
2. Understand that onco-fertility requires a multi- and interdisciplinary team
3. Begin offering information and counseling on fertility issues prior to cancer treatment
4. Take into consideration the particular problems of adolescents and young adults
5. Understand the importance of providing appropriate guidance during the entire survivorship continuum

Background Evidence

About 86,000 adolescent and young adult (AYA) cancer patients are diagnosed each year in the United States.[1] One in 46 women and one in 69 men will develop cancer before reaching 40 years of age.[1] In this young population, the chances to cure the disease are excellent: 81% of patients with cancer aged 15 to 44 years will survive the first 5 years after diagnosis.[2] These facts are changing the long-term goals for young cancer patients, and thus fertility issues are becoming more important.

Due to socioeconomic and lifestyle changes in recent decades, especially in the Western world, parenthood is increasingly being postponed to later in reproductive life. For this reason, many AYA cancer patients have not started or not fulfilled their childbearing plans at the time of diagnosis. One common side effect of oncologic therapy is partial or complete damage to the gonads, thus making it more difficult or even impossible for AYA cancer patients to have children during survivorship or reducing the fertile lifespan.

Onco-Fertility

The term *onco-fertility* was first used in 2006. This relatively new discipline, at the intersection of oncology, pediatrics, bioethics, and reproductive medicine, emerged because of the growing number of young cancer survivors facing long-term side effects of oncologic treatment on infertility and psychological functioning. Onco-fertility professionals aspire to provide exhaustive information on risks of infertility, opportunities for fertility preservation, and survivorship care.

Oncologic treatment may narrow the fertile window or lead to subfertility or infertility by damaging the gonadal tissue and the gametes or by altering the neuroendocrine axis in both men and women.[3] It is impossible to predict the individual risk of infertility resulting from oncologic therapy, as there are various related pretreatment factors like age, body mass index (BMI), reproductive health history, metabolic disease (e.g., diabetes or hypertension), history of sexually transmitted disease, and other underlying health conditions, which might influence the reproductive potential of each individual.[3] Also, a combination of different oncologic treatments, the need for multiple types of chemotherapy, or the use of high-dose, high-intensity chemotherapy may increase the risk and the reproductive impact of novel chemotherapeutics, and the impact of biological therapies remains to be elucidated. Furthermore, germ cells are very sensitive to irradiation in both men and women. The extent of gonadal damage caused by radiotherapy depends on the number of scheduled treatments, the cumulative dose, and the extent of radiation fields.

Gonadotoxic risk is stratified into four categories:

- No risk
- Low risk: less than 20% risk of infertility
- Intermediate risk: 21% to 80% risk of infertility
- High risk: 81% to 100% risk of infertility[3]

Fertility-preservation methods cannot preserve pretreatment fertility but help to overcome treatment-induced fertility impairment or infertility by preserving gametes (oocytes or sperms), parts of gonads (ovaries or testicles), or fertilized oocytes or embryos according to the circumstances and the patient's gender, underlying disease, and wishes. Also, counseling and treatment of related side effects such as pubertal delay in childhood cancer survivors, menstrual irregularities and bleeding, hormonal deficiency, and sexual dysfunctions should be adequately addressed.[3] This results in the demand for a well-organized, early referral structure between oncology units and fertility-preservation units.[4] Identification of patients' psychosocial needs is an important part of advanced onco-fertility care, including sexual health, intimate relationships, and the affordability of fertility-preservation measures.

Third-party reproductive techniques for infertile women such as egg donation or surrogate pregnancy can be offered in some countries like the United Kingdom or the United States, while in some others (e.g., Germany), such procedures are currently prohibited by law.[5] On the other hand, sperm donation can be offered for infertile men, as there are fewer legal restrictions with this procedure. Third-party reproductive techniques for infertile men, like sperm donation, are well established.[5]

Fertility and Sexual Health

A review of studies on sexual health and cancer in AYA cancer patients reported prevalence rates of sexual problems of 49% and 43% within 1 and 2 years after diagnosis, respectively.[6]

Disclosure of cancer can lead to conflicts in formation and maintenance of intimate relationships and in developing a sexual identity, together with struggles in body image and self-esteem.[6,7] Infertility was experienced as a threat to gender identity by 27% of women and 25% of men.[8] Sexual self-esteem is altered by the long-term effects of cancer therapy, leading to emotions such as anger, shock, anxiety, and frustration.[9]

Previous to their cancer diagnosis, most heterosexual persons wished to start a family in a traditional way that implied a strong desire for biologic parenthood by natural conception.[10] However, fertility issues are important irrespective of sexual orientation. Members of the LGBT (lesbian, gay, bisexual and transgender) community showed various levels of interest regarding starting a family prior to diagnosis (see also Chapter 3). They placed less importance on biologic parenthood and were considering different modalities, such as adoption.[10] Nevertheless, both heterosexual persons and members of the LGBT community felt a sense of loss and grieving when facing infertility.[10] Uncertainty develops over time; as the survivors take time to reflect on their illness, they must cope with complex, ambiguous, and unpredictable outcomes. Peate et al. reported that fertility issues become increasingly important in women with breast cancer over time, after the initial "shell shock" went away and the focus of attention and concern changed.[11]

Decisions About Fertility-Preservation Measures

Early referral to a fertility specialist facilitated the decision-making process, giving patients time to consider their options and to balance the risks and benefits.[12] Some patients felt they had not had enough time to make deliberate decisions regarding fertility preservation and felt rushed into making a decision about treatment.[10,11] Higher patient involvement in the decision-making process leads to lower decisional conflict and thus to higher satisfaction with the decision and with the healthcare provider. Most patients stated that the decision for or against fertility preservation was made after consulting a fertility specialist; thus, referral to a specialist is crucial in the decision-making process of AYA cancer patients.

Optimal Timing of Counseling

Optimal timing of counseling is important in general but especially in women because the counseling and the fertility-preservation procedures are more complex, the decision is more difficult, and some procedures in women are time-demanding, resulting in postponed initiation of oncologic treatment.[13] A timely referral is warranted, allowing both fertility specialists and patients to consider the full range of options and to value the urgency of starting cancer treatment with respect to fertility preservation.[14,15] More than 80% of women counseled reported that time pressure presented a challenge when they were trying to decide on fertility-preserving treatment options.[16] Those being referred to counseling about fertility-preserving treatment appreciated having enough time for decision-making.[17]

Nevertheless, only 61.4% of doctors, 36% of nurses, and 28.8% of allied healthcare professionals discussed the issue of fertility during the first consultation.[7] Another study showed that 29% of cancer patients had their first appointment with a fertility specialist more than 2 weeks after diagnosis, resulting in increased distress in this subgroup,[12] and some reported they were informed just before starting the oncologic therapy.[17] There were no specific factors (e.g., age, type of cancer, or parity) that were associated with late referral to a fertility specialist.[12]

Discussing Fertility Issues with Patients

Discussing fertility with cancer patients is a demanding, complex, and difficult task. The situation of newly diagnosed patients is extremely stressful and overwhelming, so it is not surprising that patients' uptake of information during a fertility counseling session may be limited. It is reported that only half of the patients remember the content of fertility issues after documented counseling by a healthcare provider, while almost one third could not remember that such a discussion had even taken place.[18] Periodic and multidisciplinary counseling, including referral to fertility specialists, can decrease patients' distress. The extent of discussions about fertility depends on the healthcare providers' knowledge about fertility risks and fertility-preservation options. Patients' perceived satisfaction with the counseling also depends on "the timing, type of information given, and level of openness of the health care professionals."[19]

Inconsistent information about cancer and fertility treatments due to inconsistency of care (i.e., seeing different clinicians) led to uncertainty about the amount and degree of possible side effects of oncologic therapy and the success of oncologic and fertility-preservation treatment. A recent study by Ussher at et. showed that 65% of women and 69% of men were satisfied with the provided counseling[17] (see Chapter 2 for details). Overall, women were more demanding regarding standards of fertility counseling and the amount of information provided and expressed more disappointment with healthcare providers, a greater level of anxiety, and a higher number of unmet needs.[13,20]

Some patients felt frustrated because of perceived lack of information and lack of clarity of the delivered information and because they did not know whom they should contact regarding fertility and menopause issues, and when they should do so.[11] AYA cancer patients stated that healthcare professionals should be proactive in regard to counseling, should offer clear and accurate explanations, and should be honest about the long-term consequences regarding fertility after cancer.[17] They stated that fertility issues should be addressed consistently and routinely,[11] and discussions about fertility should reflect the importance of this topic without healthcare providers trying to minimize the facts.[17]

Patient-centered communication implies active patient participation and patient involvement in the decision-making process. Normally, the younger the patients the more they wanted to participate in the decision-making process. Clinicians must acknowledge, understand, and appreciate patient's values, preferences, and beliefs about their illness and about health and help them to understand the actual situation, the illness, and the risks and benefits of the treatment options. AYA cancer patients reported a sense of relief when they felt they had been heard and understood by their healthcare providers and described the counseling as supportive when the provider did not try to influence their decision.[17]

Satisfaction with the amount and quality of information provided leads to better mental, physical, social, and global health-related quality of life and improved emotional and functional well-being as well as to treatment adherence.[21] Successful verbal communication as well as nonverbal behaviors can be therapeutic, helping the patient to cope with the situation, reducing anxiety and stress, and providing hope, optimism, and a sense of self-worth. It leads to access to needed care, increased patient knowledge, adherence to therapy, enhanced emotional self-management, activated social support and advocacy resources, self-efficacy and empowerment, and an improved quality of medical decisions. On the other hand, lack of information increased dissatisfaction and formal complaints and may lead to medicolegal problems. Contextual factors like the clinical setting and family and social factors may also influence the success of the communication process.

Presenting Problems

Unmet Needs Regarding Fertility and Sexual Health

Cancer survivors expressed a strong perceived connection between fertility status and sexual function: Cancer itself and/or its treatment can impact sexual desire and functioning as well as aspects associated with sexuality, such as relationships, sexual health, and fertility. There is increasing evidence that young cancer survivors have many concerns and unmet needs regarding reproductive capacity, health of progeny, desire for biologic children in the future, and their ability to manage pregnancy and raise children. Often during the transition from cancer patient to survivor, the impact of cancer and its treatment on sexuality and reproductive potential becomes apparent.

Family Building in the Survivorship Continuum and Survivorship Care

Reproductive survivorship care should be extended during the survivorship continuum, not only because of the various unmet needs of the survivors but because of possible health impairment of survivors. Unmet informational needs; unmet decision support needs; and patients' concerns about conceiving, raising children, sexual health, and financial aspects of fertility preservation were associated with greater distress and lower quality of life.[17,20] Some AYA cancer patients described possible infertility as a lifelong and life-changing experience.[22]

Assessment of reproductive potential should be offered to all cancer patients, and counseling regarding onco-fertility should be an integral part of survivorship care.[3,20,23] In childhood cancer survivors, assessment of normal physical and psychological development is crucial. Pubertal delay may be diagnosed in those with gonadal failure, and referral to a pediatric endocrinologist would be mandatory in these cases.[3]

In this context, survivors active in a large AYA advocacy organization advised newly diagnosed patients to reflect on their fertility-preservation options at the time of diagnosis, to be proactive, and to advocate for their rights regarding information about fertility impairment and fertility-preservation methods.[10] The importance of biologic parenthood may change over time.[10]

Women may worry about potential effects of a pregnancy on their health status and about potential risks to their offspring due to oncologic therapy.[17] According to published data, the offspring of cancer survivors, both men and women, do not show an increased risk of congenital malformations,[4] and the prognosis of women who become pregnant after cancer treatment is not inferior to those who did not experience a pregnancy, even in women with hormone-positive breast cancer.[4]

Survivors should be reassured that a pregnancy following oncologic treatment is usually safe for both mother and child.[4]

The relationship between cancer survivors and their partners could suffer due to parental desires, sadness and grief about future childbearing opportunities, or regrets about missed opportunities.[24] Partners may need psychological counseling referrals or couple counseling on communication and sexuality as well. Therefore, the partners' needs should be included as part of any survivorship care plans[24] (see also Chapter 7).

Barriers and Facilitators Regarding Fertility-Preservation Procedures

The Patient's Viewpoint

The decision-making process about fertility preservation is complex, difficult, and time-demanding. The decision on whether to pursue fertility preservation has to be made under tight time pressure, in a short window of opportunity. The decision has far-reaching consequences with possible rewards or regrets. Patients feel affected both by the disease itself and by the possible loss of parenting. Factors in favor of fertility preservation were the chance to retain the ability to choose in terms of future pregnancies, a solution for future infertility, and the ability to keep all options available. The wish to maintain the option for biologic parenthood was named as a factor in favor of undergoing fertility preservation by both heterosexual and LGBT persons, along with other reasons such as following the recommendations given by the medical practitioner and viewing fertility preservation as important.

Patients need individualized information about their own infertility risk and fertility potential after treatment.[13] Active involvement of a partner, a relative, or a good friend would ease the decision-making process and help to unburden the patient.

The financial costs of fertility preservation could be a major barrier for patients. As an important part of the shared decision-making process and survivorship care, financial aspects should be disclosed and less costly alternatives should be discussed early in the counseling setting. The costs of fertility preservation are significant and are higher for women (e.g., embryo, egg, or ovarian tissue cryopreservation) than for men (e.g., sperm cryopreservation). Patients may become disappointed when they discover that they cannot afford fertility treatment or that their partners are emotionally affected because they cannot access fertility preservation due to the financial costs.[25] Depending on health insurance policies, costs are not routinely covered because fertility preservation is not considered a "medically necessary" treatment for the underlying disease but rather a preventive measure for a desired outcome (i.e., having a biologic child). In Germany and other European countries there are currently efforts to clarify the cost coverage by health insurance companies.

AYA cancer patients often considered the attitudes of healthcare providers, especially oncologists, as a barrier to fertility preservation. They felt rushed into oncologic treatment without having the opportunity to discuss or decide about fertility preservation; clinicians only discussed the importance of treating the cancer, without respect to patients' wishes and fears and without respect to the long-term consequences.[17] AYA cancer patients noticed that healthcare providers seemed uncomfortable when the topic of fertility was raised, and they blamed physicians for making inaccurate assumptions about their information needs.[17] On the other hand, AYA cancer patients reported that they, too, felt uncomfortable asking about future fertility and stated that it was difficult to identify the right person to talk to on the team of healthcare providers.

Information about fertility impairment and fertility preservation should be a mandatory, integral part of cancer treatment.[13]

The Healthcare Professional's Viewpoint

Although healthcare professionals recognized the importance of fertility-preservation counseling in cancer patients, they identified a number of barriers impeding such counseling, including:

- counseling would not be appropriate given the specific stage of cancer (27%)
- counseling would be irrelevant to the patient (23%)
- lack of detailed knowledge regarding fertility-preservation methods and rates of success (63%)
- time constraints (14%)
- patient's age (over 70%)
- patient's relationship status and parenthood status.[7,10,13]

Awareness of the individual risk of fertility impairment was a facilitator or barrier with respect to fertility-preservation counseling for medical oncologists. Fifty-seven percent of women with an unknown risk level for infertility and 77% of men were not told about the risk of infertility.[13,26] Further, a low risk of infertility in first-line cancer therapy significantly reduced the likelihood of information provision, although the individual risk is unpredictable and, in case of disease recurrence, a second-line therapy might additionally diminish the chances of parenthood.

🔑 *Gender was the most important predictor for receiving information and/or counseling for fertility preservation. Men were **14 times more likely** to receive information regarding fertility preservation.*[27] Nevertheless, fertility preservation in men was more related to sexuality than in women, thus discouraging some healthcare professionals from raising the topic.[7]

Age also seemed to be an important factor in receiving fertility counseling.

🔑 *Women and men aged 30 to 39 were at increased risk of not receiving the information, even though childbearing is being increasingly postponed to later years; in contrast, younger patients were more likely to receive counseling.*[26]

Additionally, medical oncologists seemed to take into account financial factors: not being insured or being insured by the government in a U.S. population of young cancer patients was found to be a barrier to fertility counseling.[26]

Sometimes women are advised against fertility preservation because of an uncertain cancer prognosis. Among the concerns expressed by fertility specialists treating women with breast cancer were a greater or unknown risk for cancer recurrence, limited expertise related to breast cancer, and patients who lacked partners; they appreciated an information exchange with oncologists.[28]

Assessment of Fertility Issues

Indications for and Importance of Information and Counseling Regarding Fertility Preservation

🔑 *Being able to give birth is a basic human right and a human need in most social and cultural contexts.*[8] *Being deprived of the possibility of parenting a child leads to long-lasting traumatic events that can culminate in depression, lower life satisfaction, feelings of worthlessness and uselessness, and a sense of being handicapped.*[8,32]

The impact of infertility on AYA cancer survivors is longstanding and profound. Parenthood is taken for granted by most adults. Motherhood or fatherhood was described as a central goal of adult life by 25% of women and 32% of men, and a threat to fertility is seldom anticipated by AYA cancer patients.[8] In this context, fertility-preservation procedures are perceived as a "backup" in case of future infertility, an alternative to or insurance for natural conception and fertility, and a way of coping with long-term risks of oncologic therapy.[13]

Canada and Schover showed that approximately 68% of women who wanted children before a cancer diagnosis did not change their attitudes because of the diagnosis even up to 10 years after diagnosis, 15% of women experienced an increased wish for children after cancer compared to before the diagnosis, and only 17% experienced a decreased wish because of cancer.[29] Moreover, 26% of women with breast cancer reported tailoring their oncologic treatment decisions with respect to future fertility, and 1% of women chose not to receive chemotherapy or underwent mastectomies because of their fertility concerns.[30] In a European population-based study in AYA cancer patients, 80% of male patients were informed about infertility risk, 68% were counseled about fertility-preservation methods, and 54% opted for sperm banking.[27] In contrast, only 48% of women received information, 14% were counseled about fertility-preservation methods, and 2% underwent fertility-preservation methods.[27] Across the different studies, the average of those not being counseled is about 50%.[17] These data are alarming because women in particular seem to be more vulnerable than men when facing the risk of infertility[13] and because parenthood in AYA cancer survivors is reduced by 20% to 67% with respect to the normal population[31,32] and often childhood cancer survivors are diagnosed with impaired fertility as a long-term side effect of oncologic therapy. AYA cancer patients who felt abandoned and left in the dark about their possibilities and lack of information had a more challenging cancer experience.[17]

Clinicians should not assume that age is a limiting factor, as even "older" premenopausal women or women who already had children showed great interest in fertility-preservation counseling and counseling about the possibility of entering early menopause.[11] Information about possible fertility impairment at time of diagnosis was for some women "psychologically the hardest to tackle" and "the most major concern," although some women stated that the main priority, at the time of diagnosis, was deciding about oncologic treatment in order to regain their health.[11] Women more often than men experienced negative emotions regarding infertility risk, were more likely to have unmet needs regarding fertility counseling, and displayed more problems in coping with the risks of infertility.[13]

Evaluation of Fertility Before and After Cancer Treatment

It is important to assess the patient's fertility potential before starting oncologic treatment, even if this will not definitely predict the impact of therapy on his or her reproductive potential. Nevertheless, in some cases, it may help to identify a preexisting impairment of reproductive potential. In women, the preexisting reproductive potential may predict the response to some fertility-preservation methods, like ovarian stimulation, and thus may help tailor the fertility-preservation process. In women, ovarian function can be assessed by measuring the antral follicle count, anti-Müllerian hormone, and follicle-stimulating hormone (FSH) concentrations during the early follicular phase. In men, reproductive function can be evaluated by semen analysis and measuring FSH and testosterone levels.

After successful treatment of the malignancy, many young survivors are interested in their reproductive potential. In women, resumption of regular menstrual cycles does not rule out reproductive dysfunction. The fertile lifespan is shortened, even if menstruation recurs after therapy. Assessment of fertility should be carried out approximately 1 year after completion of oncologic treatment, as restoration of endocrine and reproductive function takes time.

Clinical Management

Fertility Preservation in Women

The oocyte pool is generated during fetal life and is continuously declining during the woman's lifetime as a result of intrinsic factors like the initial oocyte pool and genetically determined oocyte apoptosis. Extrinsic factors like chemotherapy and radiotherapy accelerate the decline of the remaining oocyte pool, leading to premature ovarian failure and thus infertility.

A variety of fertility-preservation methods are well established and others are still experimental or innovative. Ovarian stimulation with gonadotropins is a standard procedure and leads to multiple follicular growth. After harvesting, the oocytes are cryopreserved, either fertilized or unfertilized; both procedures are recognized as standard practice.[15,33] The cryopreserved oocytes or embryos can be stored for years to decades until retrieval. The cumulative live-birth rate after vitrification and thawing of oocytes is up to 34.0%.[34] Flexible stimulation protocols enable ovarian stimulation to be started irrespective of the day in the menstrual cycle; nevertheless, this method will lead to a delay of oncologic treatment of about 2 weeks.[35] In women with hormone-positive breast cancer, stimulation protocols using letrozole seem to be safe.[15,33] In women who need to start oncologic treatment urgently, in vitro maturation of oocytes can be offered.[3]

Another option for fertility preservation is the cryopreservation of ovarian tissue and retransplantation in case of premature ovarian failure. This procedure does not require sexual maturation and could be used in prepubertal girls after the required medical, legal, and ethical considerations.[15,33] Retransplantation can be performed in an orthotopic or heterotopic site, although to date only one live birth has been reported after heterotopic transplantation.[34] After retransplantation, a temporary restoration of ovarian function has been observed and pregnancies can be achieved either by natural conception or by assisted reproduction methods, with a cumulative live-birth rate and ongoing pregnancy rates of 57.5% and 37.7%, respectively.[36] In 63.9% of cases, ovarian function was restored at least temporarily after transplantation.[36] The procedure has some limitations in particular cancers (leukemia, neuroblastoma, Burkitt lymphoma, ovarian tumors) as they carry an increased risk of ovarian metastasis. This method is still considered experimental in the United States[33] but is already considered nonexperimental by the Sk2 guideline, which was published by the German Society of Gynecology and Obstetrics and coordinated with the German Society of Urology and the German Society of Reproductive Medicine.[35]

In women receiving pelvic irradiation, ovarian transposition and gonadal shielding are appropriate methods to reduce ovarian damage. Nevertheless, because of radiation scattering or remigration of the ovaries, these procedures have a success rate at preventing premature ovarian failure of about 50.0%.[15,33]

Conservative gynecologic surgery should considered in women with malignancies of the lower genital tract that are of low risk.[15] During recent years surgical techniques and systemic conservative treatment approaches have been developed for many cancer types, and these both provide high oncologic safety and improve body integrity.

For patients with early cervical cancer less than 2 cm in diameter and histopathologic-negative lymph nodes who desire fertility preservation without compromising oncologic outcomes, radical trachelectomy is the standard treatment. However, patients have to be counseled about decreased fertility and increased rates of abortion, prematurity, and obstetric complications.[37–39]

For patients with ovarian tumors who wish to maintain their fertility, preservation of the uterus and at least one ovary is an option for borderline tumors, unilateral ovarian carcinomas that are International Federation of Gynecology and Obstetrics (FIGO) stage IA G1 (G2), and unilateral ovarian germ-cell and sex-cord stromal tumors. Appropriate staging and counseling about a higher risk of recurrence, depending on individual risk factors, and the need for intensified follow-up must be part of this concept.[40]

For endometrial carcinoma, a conservative management plan can be considered in patients with a histologic diagnosis of grade 1 or a premalignant disease such as atypical endometrial hyperplasia. Both can be treated with oral progestin or the insertion of a levonorgestrel-containing intrauterine device.[41] Additional metformin treatment may improve overall survival in endometrial cancer and may help reverse atypical endometrial hyperplasia to normal endometrial histology.[42] Assessment of response to conservative therapies must be performed on a regular basis every 6 months with ultrasound imaging and dilatation and curettage.[41] Pregnancy is associated with a reduced risk of endometrial cancer recurrence.[43] A meta-analysis showed that the live-birth rate among women after fertility-preserving treatment for endometrial cancer was 28% and even reached 39% when assisted reproduction technologies were used.[44]

To date, there are insufficient data regarding ovarian suppression by administration of gonadotropin-releasing hormone agonists (GnRHa) during chemotherapy to preserve fertility, and the published guidelines express controversial recommendations.[33] Thus, this method could be combined with other fertility-preservation procedures and should not be used instead of established procedures for fertility preservation unless the application of GnRH is the only procedure available.[15,33] Additionally, this method will also reduce the probability of severe uterine bleeding in thrombocytopenic women due to chemotherapy and should be taken into account in this special context.[15,33]

Case Study

A 37-year-old nulligravida woman with dysmenorrhea and an ovarian mass resembling a dermoid cyst was treated by laparoscopic excision of the ovarian cyst and excision of endometriosis lesions. The histology revealed a borderline tumor of the right ovary. She was referred to our hospital for oncologic and fertility-preservation counseling. As fertility-preserving surgery is reasonable in women with borderline tumors and wish for fertility preservation, we informed her that she may have a higher risk of recurrence but without impact on long-term survival. After counseling she opted for fertility-sparing surgery and we performed a laparoscopic staging (infracolic omentectomy, peritoneal biopsies and cytology) with no sign of tumor spread. Follow-up examinations were without signs of tumor recurrence. She became pregnant 1 year after primary surgery.

Fertility Preservation in Men

Spermatogonial stem cells located on the basement membrane of seminiferous tubules start to develop with the beginning of puberty. By age 13 or 14, an effective spermatogenesis is usually established.[45] Chemotherapy and radiotherapy impair spermatogenesis. If a population of germ stem cells survives oncologic therapy, regeneration of spermatozoa may continue for years.[45] Sperm banking is an inexpensive and well-established method for fertility preservation prior to chemotherapy or radiotherapy and does not require a delay in cancer treatment. Sperm can be obtained and cryopreserved after (electro-)ejaculation or, in case of azoospermia, after testicular biopsy.[45] Sperm should be collected before treatment if possible, as sperm collected after initiation of therapy carry a risk of genetic damage.[15,33] Pregnancy success rates with frozen sperm are up to 50%.[3]

In males receiving radiation, shielding of the testicles should be offered, as even a small dosage will lead to irreversible azoospermia.[45]

Hormonal therapy in men is not beneficial and should not be recommended.[15]

Fertility-sparing surgery in males with testicular cancer should be performed in patients with low-risk cancer.[45] Prepubertal boys may benefit from testicular tissue cryopreservation.[15] If diagnosed with azoospermia later in life, retransplantation of germ stem cells may lead to resumption of spermatogonia generation.[3] Preclinical trials in this field are very promising, but this method is still highly experimental.[3,15] In prepubertal boys, cryopreservation of testicular tissue is the only option to date.[46] This method is still experimental in humans, and legal and ethical aspects should be taken into account.[46]

Professional Issues and Service Implementation

Information and Counseling

All clinicians who care for cancer patients should be able to discuss possible fertility impairment due to oncologic therapy[33] and should address this issue in all AYA cancer patients. However, 26% of doctors discussed fertility only when the patient raised it.[7] We recommend that:

🔑 ***A multidisciplinary team consisting of oncologists, fertility specialists, specialized nurses, mental health professionals, psycho-oncologists, social workers, healthcare system workers, and support groups should be in charge*** when dealing with infertility as a side effect of cancer therapy, as no single professional group has all the information and skills to successfully address the needs, worries, and insecurities related to fertility impairment due to cancer.[7,15] Fertility-preservation referral and counseling should be performed as soon as possible after the cancer diagnosis.[35,36,47]

🔑 *Communication about reproductive and sexual health, possible changes in sexuality since diagnosis, and the opportunities to experience sexual well-being despite cancer is a major task of the onco-fertility discipline.*[48]

🔑 *In general, psychosexual problems and sexual dysfunction should be proactively addressed by the physician or the psycho-oncologist, as patients or survivors often do not dare raise the topic.*[3]

Good fertility-preservation counseling should be accompanied by professional sensitivity, empathy on the part of the physician, and clarity in the information provided to avoid embarrassment.

🔑 *User-friendly information packages and decision aids may support but cannot replace good face-to-face communication and might help patients and partners to clarify their values and preferences and weigh up the different treatment possibilities and outcomes.*

Oncologists should be aware of the possible decisional conflicts due to the issue of cost coverage. Especially for AYA cancer patients who are in an early or immature state of family planning, satisfying, cost-effective choices about fertility preservation have to be discussed regarding a long-term survivorship time.

Unfortunately, there is no established training program for all healthcare professionals on how to communicate fertility-related issues. As shown in some studies, healthcare professionals in the onco-fertility field picked up their skills and insights on the job as part of their clinical practice.[7] Patients want an empathetic approach to this topic, and the support and introduction of this topic by psychological professionals might improve the disclosure.

Several guidelines recommend the referral of all patients who are interested in fertility preservation to a specialist with expertise in the field of gonadal protection for more thorough counseling and, if required and applicable, for completion of fertility-preservation procedures.[17,35,37,49–51] Standardized referral pathways have proven to be helpful.[7] Referral to a fertility specialist is crucial, as only 4% of gynecologic oncology fellows who responded a study in the United States stated that they feel capable of and comfortable counseling AYA cancer patients regarding fertility preservation.

Not all fertility specialists feel responsible for treating AYA cancer patients. A study conducted with board-certified reproductive specialists in Japan showed that only 78% of specialists would accept young breast cancer patients in their daily practice, 76% would accept married young breast cancer patients, and only 29% would accept single patients.[28] Thus, cultural factors are an important aspect for professionals to consider.

Psychological Interventions

Addressing psychosocial distress, partnership issues, or sexual problems in terms of fertility is an essential part of psycho-oncologic care of patients and survivors.

A psycho-oncologist should be a member of the interdisciplinary onco-fertility team assisting in the medical counseling process and supporting communication with patients and their partners.

Following the guidelines for distress management,[50] psychosocial distress should be assessed using a standardized tool that includes assessment across the following domains:
- *individual functions and resources (psychosocial, emotional, behavioral)*
- *social relationship (family, spouse, peers)*
- *socioeconomic situation*

For patients showing higher levels of psychological distress, psychological counseling should be offered. Psycho-oncologists may assist patients and their partners in decision-making, particularly if patients feel distressed about the potential infertility associated with cancer and its treatment or suffer from special decision conflicts. In addition, psycho-oncologists may educate patients and their partners about how to alleviate the distress by various techniques (e.g., relaxation techniques, mindfulness-based stress reduction) and help patients to improve communication with their partners. If necessary, the couple may be referred to couple psychotherapy or to a specialist in sexual therapy (see Chapter 7). If the assessment of psychosocial distress has shown elevated levels of anxiety or depression, individual psychotherapy may be indicated (see Chapter 6). In this case a referral for individual psychotherapy could be recommended to the patient.

Common Ethical Dilemmas

There are several ethical dilemmas regarding fertility preservation in cancer patients. On the one hand, clinicians have to consider whether it is reasonable to offer fertility-preservation methods to patients with an unfavorable prognosis, because it is likely that, even if they will parent a child, they will not be able to raise and support him or her. On the other hand, they have to consider whether it is appropriate to withhold information and/or medical procedures in these patients and thus deprive them of the possibility of reproduction.

Regarding third-party reproduction techniques, clinicians have to consider the frequent desire of the children to learn from whom they are descended. Oocyte donation and surrogate pregnancy is prohibited in some countries like Germany because of the great value of motherhood with respect to the genetic mother and the birth mother. Women who donate oocytes also have an increased medical risk that does not exist in men after sperm donation. Moreover, pregnant women after oocyte donation carry an increased risk for severe pregnancy complications, in both mother and child.

There is no universal answer to these questions. The solutions are different in diverse countries and localities and may change over time.

Legal Implications

Every country has complex and unique laws and regulations regarding assisted reproduction techniques with direct consequences on the procedures and approaches in AYA cancer patients and survivors seeking reproductive counseling. In case of the death of the individual, gametes are discarded according to the law in some countries. Fertilized oocytes are usually used for achieving a pregnancy only if both partners have given their agreement. Children born after third-party reproduction techniques, like sperm donation, may seek information about their genetic ancestry even decades after birth. Thus, counseling regarding fertility preservation and third-party reproduction techniques should be in line with the country's current legislation.

References

1. American Cancer Society. Cancer Facts & Figures 2019. https://www.cancer.org/research/cancer-facts-statistics/all-cancer-facts-figures/cancer-facts-figures-2019.html. Published 2019. Accessed September 2, 2019.

2. Ellison LF, Wilkins K. An update on cancer survival. *Health Rep* 2010;21(3):55–60.

3. Anazodo A, Ataman-Millhouse L, Jayasinghe Y, Woodruff TK. Oncofertility: an emerging discipline rather than a special consideration. *Pediatr Blood Cancer* 2018;65(11):e27297. doi:10.1002/pbc.27297

4. Lambertini M, Del Mastro L, Pescio MC, et al. Cancer and fertility preservation: international recommendations from an expert meeting. *BMC Med* 2016;14:1. doi:10.1186/s12916-015-0545-7

5. Fehm TN, Fleisch MKJ, eds. *Fertilitätserhalt in Der Gynäkoonkologie*. Berlin: De Gruyter, 2017.

6. Soanes L, White I. Sexuality and cancer: the experience of adolescents and young adults. *Pediatr Blood Cancer* 2018;65(12):e27396. doi:10.1002/pbc.27396

7. Ussher JM, Cummings J, Dryden A, Perz J. Talking about fertility in the context of cancer: health care professional perspectives. *Eur J Cancer Care (Engl)* 2016;25(1):99–111. doi:10.1111/ecc.12379

8. Ussher JM, Perz J. Threat of biographical disruption: the gendered construction and experience of infertility following cancer for women and men. *BMC Cancer* 2018;18. doi:10.1186/s12885-018-4172-5

9. Kenney LB, Antal Z, Ginsberg JP, et al. Improving male reproductive health after childhood, adolescent, and young adult cancer: progress and future directions for survivorship research. *J Clin Oncol* 2018;36(21):2160–2168. doi:10.1200/JCO.2017.76.3839

10. M Russell A, Galvin KM, Harper MM, Clayman ML. A comparison of heterosexual and LGBTQ cancer survivors' outlooks on relationships, family building, possible infertility, and patient-doctor fertility risk communication. *J Cancer Surviv Res Pract* 2016;10(5):935–942. doi:10.1007/s11764-016-0524-9

11. Peate M, Meiser B, Friedlander M, et al. It's now or never: fertility-related knowledge, decision-making preferences, and treatment intentions in young women with breast cancer—an Australian fertility decision aid collaborative group study. *J Clin Oncol* 2011;29(13):1670–1677. doi:10.1200/JCO.2010.31.2462

12. Kim J, Mersereau JE. Early referral makes the decision-making about fertility preservation easier: a pilot survey study of young female cancer survivors. *Support Care Cancer* 2015;23(6):1663–1667. doi:10.1007/s00520-014-2526-3

13. Armuand GM, Wettergren L, Rodriguez-Wallberg KA, Lampic C. Women more vulnerable than men when facing risk for treatment-induced infertility: a qualitative study of young adults newly diagnosed with cancer. *Acta Oncol Stockh Swed* 2015;54(2):243–252. doi:10.3109/0284186X.2014.948573

14. Dolmans M-M, Manavella DD. Recent advances in fertility preservation. *J Obstet Gynaecol Res* 2019;45(2):266–279. doi:10.1111/jog.13818

15. Loren AW, Mangu PB, Beck LN, et al. Fertility preservation for patients with cancer: American Society of Clinical Oncology clinical practice guideline update. *J Clin Oncol* 2013;31(19):2500–2510. doi:10.1200/JCO.2013.49.2678

16. Assi J, Santos J, Bonetti T, et al. Psychosocial benefits of fertility preservation for young cancer patients. *J Assist Reprod Genet* 2018;35(4):601–606. doi:10.1007/s10815-018-1131-7

17. Ussher JM, Parton C, Perz J. Need for information, honesty and respect: patient perspectives on health care professionals communication about cancer and fertility. *Reprod Health* 2018;15(1):2. doi:10.1186/s12978-017-0441-z

18. Banerjee R, Tsiapali E. Occurrence and recall rates of fertility discussions with young breast cancer patients. *Support Care Cancer* 2016;24(1):163–171. doi:10.1007/s00520-015-2758-x

19. Shen S, Zelkowitz P, Rosberger Z. Cancer and fertility: optimizing communication between patients and healthcare providers. *Curr Opin Support Palliat Care* 2019;13(1):53–58. doi:10.1097/SPC.0000000000000413

20. Benedict C, Thom B, Friedman DN, et al. Fertility information needs and concerns post-treatment contribute to lowered quality of life among young adult female cancer survivors. *Support Care Cancer* 2018;26(7):2209–2215. doi:10.1007/s00520-017-4006-z

21. Husson O, Mols F, van de Poll-Franse LV. The relation between information provision and health-related quality of life, anxiety and depression among cancer survivors: a systematic review. *Ann Oncol* 2011;22(4):761–772. doi:10.1093/annonc/mdq413

22. Frederick NN, Recklitis CJ, Blackmon JE, Bober S. Sexual dysfunction in young adult survivors of childhood cancer. *Pediatr Blood Cancer* 2016;63(9):1622–1628. doi:10.1002/pbc.26041

23. Schover LR, van der Kaaij M, van Dorst E, et al. Sexual dysfunction and infertility as late effects of cancer treatment. *Eur J Cancer Suppl* 2014;12(1):41–53. doi:10.1016/j.ejcsup.2014.03.004

24. Cohee AA, Bigatti SM, Shields CG, et al. Quality of life in partners of young and old breast cancer survivors. *Cancer Nurs* 2018;41(6):491–497. doi:10.1097/NCC.0000000000000556

25. Vogt KS, Hughes J, Wilkinson A, et al. Preserving fertility in women with cancer (PreFer): decision-making and patient-reported outcomes in women offered egg and embryo freezing prior to cancer treatment. *Psychooncology* 2018;27(12):2725–2732. doi:10.1002/pon.4866

26. Shnorhavorian M, Harlan LC, Smith AW, et al. Fertility preservation knowledge, counseling, and actions among adolescent and young adult patients with cancer: a population-based study. *Cancer* 2015;121(19):3499–3506. doi:10.1002/cncr.29328

27. Armuand GM, Rodriguez-Wallberg KA, Wettergren L, et al. Sex differences in fertility-related information received by young adult cancer survivors. *J Clin Oncol* 2012;30(17):2147–2153. doi:10.1200/JCO.2011.40.6470

28. Shimizu C, Kato T, Tamura N, et al. Perception and needs of reproductive specialists with regard to fertility preservation of young breast cancer patients. *Int J Clin Oncol* 2015;20(1):82–89. doi:10.1007/s10147-014-0676-4

29. Canada AL, Schover LR. The psychosocial impact of interrupted childbearing in long-term female cancer survivors. *Psychooncology* 2012;21(2):134–143. doi:10.1002/pon.1875

30. Ruddy KJ, Gelber SI, Tamimi RM, et al. Prospective study of fertility concerns and preservation strategies in young women with breast cancer. *J Clin Oncol* 2014;32(11):1151–1156. doi:10.1200/JCO.2013.52.8877

31. Tang S-W, Liu J, Juay L, et al. Birth rates among male cancer survivors and mortality rates among their offspring: a population-based study from Sweden. *BMC Cancer* 2016;16:196. doi:10.1186/s12885-016-2236-y

32. Stensheim H, Cvancarova M, Møller B, Fosså SD. Pregnancy after adolescent and adult cancer: a population-based matched cohort study. *Int J Cancer* 2011;129(5):1225–1236. doi:10.1002/ijc.26045

33. Oktay K, Harvey BE, Partridge AH, et al. Fertility preservation in patients with cancer: ASCO clinical practice guideline update. *J Clin Oncol* 2018;36(19):1994–2001. doi:10.1200/JCO.2018.78.1914

34. Donnez J, Dolmans M-M. Fertility preservation in women. *N Engl J Med* 2017;377(17):1657–1665. doi:10.1056/NEJMra1614676

35. Dittrich R, Kliesch S, Schüring A, et al. Fertility preservation for patients with malignant disease. Guideline of the DGGG, DGU and DGRM (S2k-Level, AWMF Registry No. 015/082, November 2017)—Recommendations and statements for girls and women. *Geburtshilfe Frauenheilkd* 2018;78(6):567–584. doi:10.1055/a-0611-5549

36. Pacheco F, Oktay K. Current success and efficiency of autologous ovarian transplantation: a meta-analysis. *Reprod Sci* 2017;24(8):1111–1120. doi:10.1177/1933719117702251

37. Feng Y, Zhang Z, Lou T, et al. The security of radical trachelectomy in the treatment of IA-IIA cervical carcinoma requires further evaluation: updated meta-analysis and trial sequential analysis. *Arch Gynecol Obstet* 2019;299(6):1525–1536. doi:10.1007/s00404-019-05141-9

38. Speiser D, Köhler C, Schneider A, Mangler M. Radical vaginal trachelectomy. *Dtsch Ärztebl Int* 2013;110(17):289–295. doi:10.3238/arztebl.2013.0289

39. Oncology guideline programme (German Cancer Society, German Cancer Aid, AWMF): S3 guideline, diagnostics, therapy and aftercare of patients with cervical cancer. September 2014. http://leitlinienprogramm-onkologie.de/Leitlinien.7.0.html. Accessed May 22, 2019.

40. Oncology guideline program (German Cancer Society, German Cancer Aid, AWMF): S3 guideline, diagnostics, therapy and aftercare of malignant ovarian tumors. March 2019. https://www.leitlinienprogramm-onkologie.de/leitlinien/ovarialkarzinom/. Accessed May 22, 2019.

41. Colombo N, Creutzberg C, Amant F, et al. ESMO-ESGO-ESTRO consensus conference on endometrial cancer: diagnosis, treatment and follow-up. *Int J Gynecol Cancer* 2016;26(1):2–30. doi:10.1097/IGC.0000000000000609

42. Meireles CG, Pereira SA, Valadares LP, et al. Effects of metformin on endometrial cancer: systematic review and meta-analysis. *Gynecol Oncol* 2017;147(1):167–180. doi:10.1016/j.ygyno.2017.07.120

43. Park J-Y, Kim D-Y, Kim J-H, et al. Long-term oncologic outcomes after fertility-sparing management using oral progestin for young women with endometrial cancer (KGOG 2002). *Eur J Cancer* 2013;49(4):868–874. doi:10.1016/j.ejca.2012.09.017

44. Koskas M, Uzan J, Luton D, et al. Prognostic factors of oncologic and reproductive outcomes in fertility-sparing management of endometrial atypical hyperplasia and adenocarcinoma: systematic review and meta-analysis. *Fertil Steril* 2014;101(3):785–794. doi:10.1016/j.fertnstert.2013.11.028

45. Rodriguez-Wallberg KA, Oktay K. Fertility preservation during cancer treatment: clinical guidelines. *Cancer Manag Res* 2014;6:105–117. doi:10.2147/CMAR.S32380

46. McDougall RJ, Gillam L, Delany C, Jayasinghe Y. Ethics of fertility preservation for prepubertal children: should clinicians offer procedures where efficacy is largely unproven? *J Med Ethics* 2018;44(1):27–31. doi:10.1136/medethics-2016-104042

47. Martinez F, International Society for Fertility Preservation–ESHRE–ASRM Expert Working Group. Update on fertility preservation from the Barcelona International Society for Fertility Preservation-ESHRE-ASRM 2015 expert meeting: indications, results and future perspectives. *Fertil Steril* 2017;108(3):407–415.e11. doi:10.1016/j.fertnstert.2017.05.024

48. Rubinsak LA, Christianson MS, Akers A, et al. Reproductive health care across the lifecourse of the female cancer patient. *Support Care Cancer* 2019;27(1):23–32. doi:10.1007/s00520-018-4360-5

49. Ethics Committee of American Society for Reproductive Medicine. Fertility preservation and reproduction in patients facing gonadotoxic therapies: a committee opinion. *Fertil Steril* 2013;100(5):1224–1231. doi:10.1016/j.fertnstert.2013.08.041

50. National Comprehensive Cancer Network. Guidelines, adolescent and young adult (AYA) oncology. October 2018. www.nccn.org

Further Reading

Quinn GP, Vadaparampil ST, eds. *Reproductive Health and Cancer in Adolescents and Young Adults*. Advances in Experimental Medicine and Biology, Vol. 732. Springer Science and Business Media, 2012.

Woodruff TK, Snyder KA, eds. *Oncofertility: Fertility Preservation for Cancer Survivors*. Cancer Treatment and Research, Vol. 138. Springer US, 2007.

Woodruff TK, Zoloth L, Camp-Engelstein L, Rodriguez S, eds. *Oncofertility: Ethical, Legal, Social, and Medical Perspectives*. Cancer Treatment and Research, Vol. 156. Springer US, 2010.

Chapter 2

Provision of Sexual Health Support

Jane M. Ussher, Alexandra Hawkey, and Janette Perz

Learning Objectives

After reading this chapter the clinician will be able to:

1. Understand how cancer treatment may affect patients' sexual health and well-being
2. Have awareness of differences in the emotional/sexual/intimacy needs of people with cancer according to tumor site
3. Provide guidance for healthcare professionals in addressing issues associated with cancer and sexuality in the clinical context
4. Examine barriers to communication about sexual health concerns from the perspective of patients, their partners, and healthcare professionals

Background Evidence

Changes to sexuality and intimacy are a common consequence of cancer and cancer treatment. Such changes are multifaceted and are linked with a range of negative physical and emotional outcomes for both people with cancer and their partners as well as changes to roles and intimate relationships.[1] It is estimated that 50% of people with cancers of gonads, reproductive organs, and pelvic tissues will experience negative changes to their sexual functioning, and over 25% to 40% of people with other forms of cancer will also experience such changes.[2] Sexual difficulties following cancer are primarily the result of the effects of cancer treatments rather than the disease itself. Cancer treatment, including surgery, radiation therapy, chemotherapy, and hormone therapy, can result in both direct and indirect physical changes to sexual functioning. The impact of such changes depends on the modalities of treatment or treatment combinations and may be temporary or may last for many years after successful treatment.

For women, the focus of research and clinical guidelines has been on the impact of treatments for gynecologic or breast cancer, which can result in anatomic changes (e.g., vaginal shortening or reduced vaginal elasticity, pelvic nerve damage, clitoris removal, vaginal stenosis, and fistula formation) and physical changes (e.g., decreased bodily function, fatigue, dyspareunia, vaginal dryness, infertility, and postcoital vaginal bleeding).[3,4] Negative body image or feelings of sexual unattractiveness, concern about weight gain or loss, loss of femininity, and alterations to the sexual self can exacerbate the impact of these physical changes.[5] In combination, this can result in changes to women's sexual response, including changes to desire, orgasm, arousal, vaginal lubrication, genital swelling, and genital sensitivity, leading to decreased frequency of sex and lack of sexual pleasure or satisfaction.

Research and clinical guidelines on men's sexuality after cancer has primarily focused on prostate and testicular cancer.[6] Men with prostate cancer have reported that hormone therapy is like "chemical castration," resulting in erectile dysfunction, diminished genital size, weight gain, urinary incontinence, and bodily feminization. Other treatments result in loss of sexual desire, erotic dreams, and sexual fantasies; decreased orgasmic sensation; and bowel and urinary incontinence. Similarly, following surgery for testicular cancer, men have reported reductions in sexual functioning and enjoyment, fertility concerns, and negative body image. Rectal cancer has also been associated with reductions in sexual functioning for both women and men.

Sexual changes can also result from cancers of nonreproductive organs, such as colorectal, colon, head and neck, bladder, lymphatic, and lung cancers.[7] Women and men can experience a reduction in sexual interest and sexual activity, changes to body image and feelings of sexual competency, and sexual dysfunction and alterations to sexual self-esteem.[1] Adult survivors of childhood cancer, across a range of cancer types and treatments, also report sexual difficulties and concerns.

A loss of sexual function and physical changes to the body as a consequence of cancer treatment may be associated with anxiety, depression, lowered quality of life, loss of self-esteem, and relational conflict.[1] Conversely, maintaining intimacy and sex can help reduce emotional distress related to cancer, improve psychosocial well-being and quality of life, and facilitate adjustment to a cancer diagnosis. There is some evidence that men are more distressed than women by changes in sexual functioning after cancer[8] and that gay and bisexual men have higher rates of distress than heterosexual men.[9] Conversely, a positive couple relationship, and couple communication about sexual concerns, is associated with sexual satisfaction and higher levels of sexual functioning after cancer treatment.[1] Good couple communication has also been reported to be associated with successful renegotiation of sexual practices after cancer.[10]

It is important to address sexual difficulties in the context of cancer and cancer treatment. There is evidence that people with cancer and their partners report the need for information about sexuality after cancer treatment from health professionals; however, such information provision is often inadequate or absent.[11] Particular areas of unmet need include open communication about postcancer physical and sexual changes, effects of treatments on sexuality and body image, changes to intimate relationships, and psychological support. Absence of communication and information can leave people with cancer and their partners feeling that they are sexually "abnormal," unprepared for the sexual side effects of cancer and treatments, lacking in knowledge about the cause and duration of their sexual problems, depressed, or disappointed with health professionals. In contrast, being provided with information and being included in an open discussion about sexuality can alleviate anxiety around postcancer sexual changes, assist people with cancer to discuss sexuality with their partner and develop strategies to address sexual changes, minimize the negative impact on intimate relationships, and enhance quality of life.[12]

To encourage patient–clinician communication about sexuality after cancer, a range of clinical practice guidelines and sexual communication models such as PLISSIT[13] and BETTER[14] have been developed (outlined in detail below). These guidelines and models concur in advocating discussion of sexuality with all cancer patients and their partners, provide models of how such discussion should take place, and offer recommendations for when referral for specialist intervention is appropriate. However, research has consistently identified a range of barriers to health professional information provision and communication about sexuality in the context of cancer. This includes personal and structural constraints, sociocultural constructions of sexuality and illness adopted by clinicians, and reluctance to discuss sexuality with particular demographic groups, including older people, those from culturally diverse backgrounds, and lesbian, gay, bisexual, transsexual, queer or intersex (LGBTQI) people.[15]

This chapter will focus on cancer treatment side effects and their impact on sexuality and sexual functioning, risk factors for experiencing sexual difficulties, and the clinical management of sexual changes. We will also address barriers to effective communication about sexuality and sexual changes and explore specific cultural or ethical challenges when providing support to people with cancer and their partners. We then examine clinical management of problems and strategies for effective communication with patients and their partners about sexual concerns.

Presenting Problems

Impact of Cancer Treatment on Sexual Functioning and Well-Being

Surgery
Different forms of surgery affect sexuality and intimacy in different ways. Some forms of surgery remove parts of or whole sex organs, directly affecting sexual functioning. Other forms of surgery, such as bowel or bladder surgery, may produce a stoma or cause incontinence, with negative implications for sexuality, intimacy, and self-image. Surgery can also cause damage to nerves, which may affect sexual functioning, sensation, and pleasure. The impacts of surgery also differ according to tumor type and between men and women, as illustrated in Table 2.1 in the case of pelvic surgery.

Radiation Therapy
Radiation to the pelvic area can cause a number of changes to sexual functioning for both men and women. It may decrease bladder capacity, resulting

Table 2.1 Impacts of Surgery on Sexuality

Women	Potential Impacts
Breast surgery	Loss of breast and nipple sensation; mastectomy may affect sexual arousal; body image concerns; impacts to sense of female identity; concerns about partner reactions
Hysterectomy	Shortening of vagina; changes to orgasm; infertility
Oophorectomy	Bilateral oophorectomy may result in early menopause and infertility; hormonal changes may result in vaginal dryness and tightening
Vulvectomy	Altered appearance and sensation to genital area; changes to orgasm, particularly if clitoris is removed
Vaginal surgery	Dyspareunia due to scar tissue; vaginal dryness, tightness, and shortening
Men	**Potential Impacts**
Abdomen/pelvic surgery	Surgery for bowel, bladder, or prostate cancer may cause temporary or long-lasting erectile dysfunction
Prostatectomy	Erection difficulties; lack of ejaculate; retrograde ejaculation; urine incontinence during intercourse or orgasm; loss of pleasure; pain during orgasm
Orchiectomy (removal of testicles)	Changes to scrotum appearance, infertility with bilateral orchiectomy
Penectomy	Changes in penis size and shape; erectile difficulties
Abdominoperineal resection (removal of anus)	Loss of erogenous zone; inability to have penetrative sex for men who have sex with men

in problems with urinary frequency, urgency, and incontinence. Inflammation from radiation can cause disruptions to the bowel, including bloody mucus and diarrhea, which may be temporary or long-lasting.

For women, radiation to the pelvic region may affect the ovaries, interrupting hormone production. This can cause a disruption to the menstrual cycle, with implications for fertility. It may induce urogenital symptoms such as a dry or itchy vagina. Radiation can also cause skin fibrosis and vaginal narrowing and shortening, which may result in altered sensation and dyspareunia.

Radiation treatment is frequently used to treat prostate, bladder, and rectal cancers in men. This can result in damage to the blood vessels and nerves that facilitate erections, resulting in temporary or permanent erectile dysfunction. Radiation can cause inflammation to the urethra, meaning ejaculation may be painful for some men in the weeks following treatment. It may also cause a reduction in sperm production, negatively impacting fertility.

Chemotherapy

Side effects of chemotherapy depend on the specific drugs given. Often they include nausea, vomiting, diarrhea, hair loss, constipation, and mouth ulcers, all of which may decrease libido. Further, chemotherapy may directly affect sex hormones, resulting in low sexual desire. For women, chemotherapy may cause a decrease in ovarian hormones, meaning menstruation may become irregular. It may bring on menopause, which can be temporary or permanent.

Premature menopause due to cancer treatment is a significant quality-of-life issue associated with infertility, impaired sexual functioning, and challenges in managing menopausal changes such as vaginal dryness and hot flushes. For men, chemotherapy can lower sperm production, in addition to sperm motility, resulting in temporary or permanent infertility.

Hormone Therapy

Endocrine or androgen deprivation therapy (ADT) may affect sexuality. Drugs used to treat breast cancer such as tamoxifen, and aromatase inhibitors (anastrozole, letrozole, and exemestane) for some women, can result in vaginal dryness or discharge, dyspareunia, hot flushes, weight gain, reduced sexual desire, night sweats, changes in moods, and urinary problems. They may increase the risk of endometrial cancer, requiring regular gynecologic checkups. For men with prostate cancer who receive ADT, reported side effects include fatigue, low sexual desire, weight gain, hot flushes, erectile problems, breast growth and tenderness, depression, and osteoporosis.

Emotional Consequences of Sexual Changes Due to Cancer and Cancer Treatment

Psychological distress associated with cancer, as well as changes to sexuality in the context of cancer treatment, can lead to anxiety, depression, distress, and negative perceptions of sexual identity and body image. Socially constructed discourses surrounding gender and sexuality shape women's and men's experiences of their sexual well-being following cancer treatment. For example, women may describe feeling a loss of womanhood and femininity, particularly with the removal of, or changes to, their reproductive organs. Many studies report that women with a diagnosis of gynecologic cancer experience fear and anxiety surrounding sexual function, including concerns about sexual pain and the ability to perform. Fears surrounding a lack of sexual activity following cancer or inability to meet the sexual needs of one's partner, in addition to worries about sexual interactions for future relationships, have also been reported. Worries about injury during sex, the fear of cancer recurrence, and distress related to infertility can also affect women's psychosexual well-being.

For heterosexual men, particularly those with prostate cancer, distress surrounding a lack of physical or emotional sexual response to women and diminished feelings of manhood due to a loss in sexual functioning are commonly reported. Men also report anxiety related to sexual performance with their partners and fear that they will be unable to sexually satisfy their partner following changes associated with cancer treatment. Psychological interventions aimed at reducing distress and improving quality of life after cancer should include a component on sexual well-being, and sexual interventions should incorporate components on psychological and relational functioning.

Relationship Consequences of Changes to Sexuality

Changes in sexual health following cancer treatment can have an impact on couple relationships. It can be difficult to maintain previous roles and expectations in the face of physical changes or the inability or unwillingness of one or both partners to engage sexually. Maintaining intimacy or a sexual relationship within a couple can be difficult if one person is positioned as a patient and the other as a caregiver. Individuals can become emotionally distant from each other if sexual intimacy is reduced or if there are perceived changes in the partner's level of interest in sexual activity. Communication difficulties are common, with both partners feeling unable to discuss the changes to their sexual relationship. Partners can have a negative reaction to bodily changes following cancer treatment, and those with cancer can fear negative reactions to their body. For those who are not in a relationship, there can also be concerns about the effect of treatment on future intimate partner relationships.

Clinical Management

Provision of General Sexual Health Information and Advice: The PLISSIT Model

In order to encourage patient–clinician communication about sexuality after cancer, a range of clinical practice guidelines and sexual communication models have been developed. These guidelines and models concur in advocating discussion of sexuality with all cancer patients and their partners, provide models of how such discussion should take place, and recommendations for when referral for specialist intervention is appropriate.

The PLISSIT model,[13] which advocates four levels of intervention— *Permission, Limited Information, Specific Suggestions*, and *Intensive Therapy*—is widely recommended as a framework for providing general information and support for people with sexual concerns or difficulties. It is effective in guiding communication and support in the context of sexual changes that result from cancer or cancer treatment. This model encourages health professionals to engage in the discussion of sexual changes at various levels of increasing intensity, represented visually as an inverted pyramid (Figure 2.1).

Permission

The model starts with challenging the misconception that sexuality is "frivolous" during cancer by raising the issue with all patients and "giving permission" for couples to talk about sex and be sexually intimate. Many patients and their partners feel embarrassed to discuss sexuality with a clinician, or within the couple relationship, and will not raise the issue if the clinician does not raise it. Permission to discuss sexuality after cancer can raise awareness of sexual concerns, act to normalize sexual changes, reassure people that they are not abnormal, and educate them that there are solutions to many problems. Box 2.1 provides extracts from interviews with cancer patients and their partners to illustrate the impact and importance of this permission giving.[12]

Limited Information

The second stage of the model avoids the risk of providing unwanted or irrelevant interventions to patients and their partners by encouraging the provision of "limited information," in written form or through online resources, only to those who want it. There is evidence that although some individuals

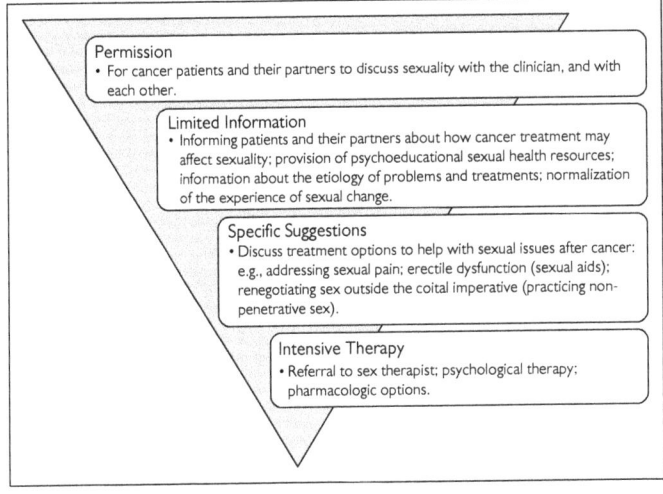

Figure 2.1 PLISSIT model of sexual information and support in the context of cancer

---

Box 2.1 Impact of Permission to Talk About Sex

Increasing Awareness

"Having the issue of sex raised with us increased our awareness of both our sexual needs and made me think about it more. It brought sex into focus and put it on the agenda." (Angela, 48, colorectal cancer survivor)

"I think people find sexuality a difficult thing to talk about, or an embarrassing thing to talk about, or it's very low on your list of priorities when you are undergoing chronic illness. But, there's a reminder there that it shouldn't be that sort of threatening, that it an important part of an ongoing, loving relationship you have with somebody, be it your wife or partner or lover or whatever it is." (Simon, 53, sarcoma survivor)

Opening Up Communication About Sex

"There were still a few things that I hadn't yet got around to asking my wife, but when the nurse asked us about sex, it actually saved me from having to ask, or when I did ask, it was more around, 'So is this what happened with you?'" (Jason, 35, husband of a woman with non-Hodgkin lymphoma)

"We had a normal and good sex life, but talking to the doctor helped us to talk a little more about sexual things." (David, 63, prostate cancer survivor)

Normalizing Sexual Changes

"I found the recognition that there are problems with sexuality with cancer very helpful. It is better to be in a boat with others rather than trying to paddle alone through rough waters." (Emma, 68, breast cancer survivor)

with cancer prefer face-to-face consultation sessions about sexual changes, others prefer written or online information, or a combination of the two, with the need for face-to-face consultations being greater close to diagnosis and the preference for written information increasing over time. Box 2.2 gives examples of how having information has assisted communication and well-being for people with cancer.[12]

Specific Suggestions

If required, clinicians can provide "specific suggestions" related to the adjustment to sexual changes and expansion of sexual repertoires, including redefining sex as "not just penetration"; embracing nongenital intimacy; changing sexual positions; or using sexual enhancement products, such as sex aids, lubricant, or penile pumps. The primary aim of providing information and education to address sexual changes after cancer may not be to return individuals to the level of sexual functioning that they enjoyed before cancer; this can be difficult for many to achieve, particularly when clinical levels of sexual difficulties are reported. A focus on improving intimacy,

---

Box 2.2 Impact of "Limited Information" About Sexual Changes After Cancer: Booklets and Online Information Provision

Assisting with Communication About Specific Sexual Concerns

"Having written information about sex and cancer was very helpful. You could make your partner aware and just say, 'Look, you know, there's something for you to read if you want a relationship with me. These are my issues. Or some of my issues.'" (Boris, 61, prostate cancer survivor)

"I had just gone into a new relationship about 8 months ago and this person wasn't with me when I was going to my treatment, so having the booklet about sex and cancer was just a really good springboard for me to open up discussion with him about where I'm at sexually." (Zoe, 48, breast cancer survivor)

Assisting with Seeking Help for Sexual Problems

"Having the information booklet about sex and cancer helped with discussing sex with my oncologist. I also went to my GP for creams and soreness, which helped a bit." (India, 51, breast cancer survivor)

"Having information online helped me to ask for penile injections. I knew what they were and who to go to"; "It meant I asked for help with my erectile dysfunction, which finally led to my having a prosthesis." (Men with prostate cancer)

Reducing Distress About Sexual Changes

"Reading about sexual changes after cancer meant I didn't feel so guilty about lack of sex, and not wanting sex. I had a greater sense of not worrying about it, as I realized that there is nothing shameful and embarrassing about the condition. I wish I'd had this information at the beginning of treatment." (Duncan, 57, lung cancer survivor)

sexual flexibility, and renegotiation of sex is a more achievable outcome for many individuals.

Many heterosexual couples cease engaging in any sexual activity if coital sex is not possible, as sexual intercourse is conceptualized as "real sex," a phenomenon described as the "coital imperative." Noncoital sexual expression and intimacy should not be positioned as a poor substitute for, or inferior to, "real sex." People who believe that sex equals penetrative intercourse have been found to be less likely to explore noncoital intimacy or sexual practices, and more likely to report that provision of information and support is not useful for them. For those who can effectively use medical and other assistive aids, this is not problematic. However, assistive aids are not effective for many individuals, and the absence of exploration of noncoital sexual practices can lead to sexual abstinence, with negative consequences for well-being and couple relationships.

Box 2.3 illustrates ways in which couples have successfully renegotiated sex after cancer.[10]

Intensive Therapy

If there is a desire for "intensive sexual therapy" or medical intervention, clinicians can refer patients to specialists for appropriate support, such as sex

---

Box 2.3 Impact of Specific Suggestions: How to Renegotiate Sex After Cancer

Redefining Sex (as "not just penetration"—exploring noncoital sexual practices, including masturbation, mutual genital touching, oral sex, shared sexual fantasies)

"I can't get an erection but I think we have as nearly as good a sex life as before the operation. So you know, in terms of, it depends what, how hooked you are on penetration." (Phil, 68, prostate cancer survivor)

"Learning different techniques on how to do hand jobs, and just things like that is interesting and fun, and our sex life is very good." (Ruby, 49, ovarian cancer survivor)

Embracing Intimacy (cuddling, kissing, nongenital touching, massage, spending time together, caring, or talking)

"The discussion of intimacy as different to sexuality was very good, and encouraged the touching and listening. We were reminded that you can have intimacy that doesn't involve sex. And my husband seemed somewhat relieved to just kiss and cuddle." (Grace, 65, wife of man with prostate cancer)

Using Sexual or Medical Aids (vibrators, lubricant, dilators, erectile dysfunction medications, penile injections, pumps, and implants)

"We've had a veil lifted and feel more confident in exploring sex toys. Now we know it's OK if we do this, next time we pass one or go near a sex shop we would most likely enter without feeling shy." (John, 72, prostate cancer survivor)

therapists or relationship therapists (Box 2.4). This decision may be made by the patient and partner, who ask for more intensive support than is available from a clinician working in oncology. Or the decision may be made by the oncology medical, nursing, or allied health clinician, based on assessment of the nature and magnitude of the sexual concerns and the clinician's ability to address them. There are a number of instances where provision of basic information about sexual changes is not sufficient and referral for specialist support may be warranted. Provision of limited information and specific suggestions may not be adequate in addressing the sexual concerns of the patient and partner. There may be a high level of distress that needs to be addressed within a more intensive and complex intervention.

Differential diagnosis is important and may result in a referral for intensive therapy. Sexual difficulties may result from another acute or chronic health condition experienced by the patient or partner, such as heart disease, diabetes, or major depression. Sexual difficulties may be a longstanding problem that could have been exacerbated by the cancer diagnosis and treatment. Relationship difficulties, which may be longstanding or may have arisen in the context of cancer, may also result in sexual problems. Difficulties in sexual functioning may also reflect the normal aging process; erectile difficulties, vaginal dryness, and reduced libido are common in older people.

Full assessment of the history and nature of the sexual difficulties, their impact on the couple, and any other health conditions is the first step in assessing whether referral for intensive therapy is needed and the appropriate avenue for referral. If the focus of concern is sexual functioning, a sex therapist, possibly alongside a practitioner who can facilitate biomedical aids, would be the appropriate referral. Couple or relationship difficulties could also be addressed by a relationship counselor or by a psychologist specializing in couple therapy. High levels of psychological distress should be addressed by a psychologist.

Box 2.4 Intensive Therapy: What It Is and When to Refer

Intensive therapy: sex therapy, couple counseling, psychological therapy, cancer-specific interventions focusing on sexual health

Biomedical interventions to address sexual functioning also need specialist or medical referral: penile implants or injections, erectile dysfunction medications such as sildenafil (Viagra) or tadalafil (Cialis), vaginal dilators, and hormonal creams

When to refer:
1. Information and specific suggestions are insufficient to address the patient's sexual concerns.
2. High levels of distress are associated with sexual changes.
3. Couple or relationship difficulties exist that are associated with distress.
4. A comorbid health condition is present that exacerbates sexual concerns or needs specialist referral.

Effectiveness of Sexual Health Information and Support

There is evidence that sexual health information and support in a cancer context provided within a PLISSIT model can improve sexual satisfaction and have a positive effect on self-efficacy for enjoying intimacy.[12] Cancer patients and their partners report that sex is legitimated as a concern, that problems are normalized, and that they can successfully renegotiate sexual practices to include noncoital intimacy. This is a result of people feeling more confident about talking about sex with their partner as well as exploring "flexible" sexual practices such as touching, kissing, and using sex toys.

The ability to develop "flexible" sexual practices or to "renegotiate" sexual behavior to include noncoital sex and nongenital intimacy[10] can allow couples to maintain sexual activity and intimacy after cancer. There is evidence that gay and bisexual men, and lesbian women, are more open to sexual renegotiation after cancer, as their sexual practices are not tied to coital sex (see Chapter 3). However, many heterosexual couples also report that renegotiated sexual practices can be experienced as positive and enjoyable, and even in some instances as an improvement over precancer sexual intimacy and pleasure.

More intensive psychological interventions that offer a number of sessions of one-to-one intervention, drawing on principles of sex therapy and psychological therapy, can also have a positive effect on sexual health and sexual functioning. There is also evidence that such interventions have a positive impact on psychological well-being. There is evidence that psychological interventions for sexual difficulties after cancer are more effective when they are couple-based, or when partners engage with the process by completing homework activities. This suggests that clinicians should emphasize couple communication and exploration of sexual changes, regardless of whether the intervention is individual- or couple-based (see Chapter 5 in this book).

Case Study: Addressing Changes in Sexual Functioning and Relationship Difficulties After Cancer

David is a 50-year-old who has been treated for prostate cancer. His wife, Amy, is 47, and they have been together for over 20 years. They had not expected the changes to erectile functioning after David had a prostatectomy and were devastated about not being able to engage in sexual intercourse. Sex had been a central part of their life together, and they now had no sexual intimacy at all. David was too embarrassed and ashamed to talk to Amy about his feelings of loss, and Amy didn't raise the issue of sex with David as she didn't want to make him feel bad. Both felt very alone and sexually frustrated and missed the intimacy they had previously shared.

In a posttreatment follow-up consultation, a new oncology registrar asked David how he was coping sexually and if he had noticed changes. David was relieved to be able to talk about his concerns and how the loss of erectile functioning made him feel. Amy was in the consultation and was able to say that she missed cuddling and kissing, as well as having sex. The registrar gave David and Amy a booklet to read about sexual changes after cancer and suggested they read through it together. They could discuss it with him at the next meeting if they wanted to.

At the next consultation, the registrar asked David and Amy if they had read the booklet. They said that they had found it helpful to know the causes of their sexual difficulties but were still stuck in terms of sexual intimacy. The registrar suggested that they talk to each other about how they were feeling and think about ways in which they could still be intimate, even if they couldn't have intercourse any more. He turned to the pages in the booklet that talked about sexual activities other than intercourse, such as oral sex or mutual masturbation. He suggested that massage, cuddling, and other forms of touch could be very pleasurable. He also talked to David about whether he was interested in exploring options to regain erectile functioning and said he could try tadalafil (Cialis) as well as a vacuum pump. David said he was interested, and the registrar said he would refer the couple to a colleague who specialized in medical interventions for erectile difficulties. He also told them that, if they were interested, he could refer them to a psychologist who specialized in sexual health issues, who would work with them in more depth in relation to their sexual concerns.

Professional Issues and Service Implementation

Communication Issues

There is evidence that people with cancer and their partners want information about sexual health after cancer from healthcare professionals. However, such information provision is often inadequate or absent. When sexuality is raised by healthcare professionals, the focus is often on bodily changes, such as erectile functioning, or vaginal dryness, and the impact on coital sex. This narrow focus or absence of information or communication can leave people with cancer and their partners struggling to cope with changes to sexuality, feeling let down by healthcare professionals, or feeling as though their sexual needs and concerns are not legitimate. Individuals are also unprepared for the sexual side effects of cancer and treatments and lack knowledge about the cause and duration of their sexual problems. This can result in depression, or disappointment with health professionals. Barriers to communication about sex from the perspective of patients, their partners, and healthcare professionals are summarized in Box 2.5.[11,15]

Barriers to Communication About Sexual Health and Cancer

Healthcare Professional Perspectives

Although many health professionals recognize that sexual health as an important topic of discussion in the context of cancer, this does not always translate into practice. A number of personal, patient-centered, and situational barriers that prevent health professionals from discussing sexuality and meeting the sexual information needs of people with cancer and partners have been identified.

- *Personal factors* include lacking knowledge or confidence in discussing sex with patients, feeling ill equipped to provide answers about sexual

> **Box 2.5 Barriers to Communication About Sex from the Perspective of Patients, Partners, and Healthcare Professionals**
>
> *Patients/Partners*
> Waiting for clinician to raise the issue; embarrassment; shame; feeling abnormal; unsympathetic response from healthcare professional; LGBTQI and not "out" to clinician; perception of care as heteronormative; cultural barriers to discussing sex; gender of clinician (e.g., women not discussing sex with a man)
>
> *Healthcare Professional Barriers*
> **Personal**: Lack of knowledge, confidence, or comfort in discussing sex after cancer; embarrassment; discomfort with particular groups of patients (e.g., LGBTQI, culturally diverse people)
> **Structural**: Time pressure; lack of privacy in clinical setting; seeing sexual health as someone else's concern; clinical culture as oriented toward cure; sex silenced in clinical care
> **Patient-centered**: Survival is prioritized over sexual health; sex is not seen as an issue for some people (e.g., older, younger, single people, non-sexual cancer patients, or those in palliative care)

concerns, and feeling embarrassed or uncomfortable in discussing sexual issues.

- *Patient-centered factors* include the belief that some patients are asexual or not interested in sexuality and the belief that discussing sexuality is too risky or inappropriate to raise with some patients. This includes single, older, LGBTQI, and culturally diverse people, or people who are considered "too sick." The presence of a partner, family member, or friend may also impede discussion.
- *Structural factors* include the absence of a private space for discussion, absence of time, the belief that discussion of sexuality with patients is someone else's responsibility, and lack of referral sources. It has also been suggested that some health professionals work dominantly within a clinical culture that is more "cure-oriented" than "care-oriented," with sexual concerns not easily "cured."

Box 2.6 provides healthcare practitioners' accounts of barriers to communication about sex in the context of cancer.[15]

Patient Perspectives

There is evidence that people with cancer and their partners tend not to initiate a discussion of sexual health concerns unless health professionals provide the opportunity. Many believe that if sexuality were important, health professionals would have raised the issue with them. As they trust "the expert," this reinforces the view that sexual issues are not legitimate or important in the context of cancer. Equally, many patients are shy or embarrassed or do not know how to raise sexual concerns. They may feel ashamed of

Box 2.6 Barriers to Communication About Sexual Health in the Context of Cancer: Accounts from Healthcare Professionals

Lack of Knowledge or Training

"I feel that it's something that's swept under the carpet and if the clients bring it up that's OK, we address it, but we really are not as equipped as we'd like to be." (Olive, social worker, gynecology)

"I don't feel trained or experienced enough to be able to provide factual information or sex therapy for people." (Nancy, nurse, general oncology)

Time and Privacy Issues

"It depends on how many patients we've got to see in a short period of time. Broaching the subject of sex will definitely double your consultation time." (Hope, general practitioner)

"One of the problems on the wards is the fact that the curtains are very thin. If someone asked a patient about their sexual function and it was a four-bedded room you'll know damn well everyone is listening for the answer." (Gail, doctor, general oncology)

Focusing on Patient Survival

"Sexuality gets pushed into the background because in oncology you tend to have a run of tragic cases and the sexuality side of things just gets pushed to the background in those patients because you're just struggling to keep them alive." (Andrew, oncologist, gynecology)

Not My Responsibility

"I think it should come from the doctors because they have a much more ongoing and intimate relationship with the patient." (Colleen, nurse, general oncology)

"'I think it probably is part of the role of the clinical psychologist who's looking at psychological issues, of dealing with the cancer, to bring issues of sexuality up." (Mark, doctor, hematology)

Patient-Related Barriers

"With quite elderly patients, I'm always surprised at how many say to me, 'Oh, yeah, well, we are reasonably sexually active' . . . you know, even people in their 70s, and you think 'Oh, gosh,' you know—'Don't shoot myself in the foot and say something stupid.'" (Maree, doctor, general oncology)

"I'd feel like I couldn't bring it up with someone who didn't have a significant other." (Michele, social worker, hematology)

"It's not something I go out to ask everyone about routinely unless they are specifically a GYN or a prostate patient." (Helen, doctor, general oncology)

changes to their sexual function, feel that they are abnormal, or not realize that there are solutions to their concerns. If concerns are addressed with a clinician, often tentatively, the absence of a positive response can shut down further communication.

- For individuals from cultural groups where discussion of sex is taboo, raising such concerns can be more difficult.
- Discussion of sexuality with a healthcare professional of a different gender from the patient (e.g., a woman discussing sex with a male clinician) may be more difficult, embarrassing, or taboo.
- Adolescents and young adults may be reluctant to discuss sexual health concerns if their parents are present in clinical consultations.
- For LGBTQI patients, previous experience of negative reactions from healthcare professionals to disclosure of sexuality or gender diversity, or fear of a negative reaction to disclosure, can also act as an inhibitor.
- Finally, not all patients want to discuss sexual issues with a healthcare professional. They may prefer to locate information themselves, in a written or online format.

Box 2.7 provides patients' accounts of barriers to communication about sex in the context of cancer.[11]

Box 2.7 Barriers to Communication About Sexual Health in the Context of Cancer: Patient Accounts

Waiting for Clinicians to Raise the Issue
"Sex was not given any significance by my oncologist—maybe they could have suggested resources instead of me having to find them."

"I am in my mid-50s. Not a single health professional I have ever consulted throughout my life has raised sexuality issues. No questions. No acknowledgment."

Embarrassment in Raising the Discussion
"It really took me a lot to go in and talk to my doctor about having a sexual problem. I even said to her, 'Oh, my God, I've done it,' you know. I said, 'I've actually come in and spoken about it.' And I felt really good because it just broke that barrier. She could then start to help me find solutions." (Tom, 65, pancreatic cancer)

Feeling Sex Was Not a Legitimate Concern
"My GP, I talked to him more about the fact that I'd gone through a premature menopause. He shrugged his shoulders and he said, 'Well, that's to be expected,' and I asked for something and he gave me Ovestin cream. There was no other comment made and I was never asked about it again, even though sex was excruciatingly painful." (Helen, 64, colorectal cancer)

Groups at Risk of Not Receiving Cancer-Related Sexual Health Information and Support

Partners

There is evidence that partners are more likely to be absent from any discussion about sexuality and cancer. This is problematic in the light of research showing that intimate partners have reported worsened sexual functioning after cancer, independent of the survivor's experience. Indeed, partners have reported experiencing a range of sexual changes after cancer, including:

- decreased frequency of sex
- complete cessation of sexual relationship
- tiredness, lack of sexual spontaneity
- reluctance to initiate sex
- repositioning of their partner as an asexual sick patient.[16]

These changes can leave partners feeling frustrated, sad, and unable to assist in the sexual and emotional health of their partner with cancer.

Although there is evidence to suggest that the majority of partners receive some form of information from patients with whom they are in an intimate relationship, it is important to bear in mind that the informational needs of patients and partners are not necessarily identical in content and quantity, and that patients tend to be more satisfied with information received than partners. In addition, the idea that partners should have to rely on patients for information assumes that patients are being provided with the opportunity to discuss sexuality with a health professional in the first instance. As outlined above, this is often not the case. It also assumes that patients with cancer will pass this information on; however, the passing on of information between partners is contingent on the level of couple communication, meaning that those lacking in couple communication may be especially likely to have unmet sexual needs.

Patients with Cancers Outside the Sexual or Reproductive Organs

People with cancer and partners living with a cancer that is not of the sexual or reproductive organs are less likely to report having a discussion of sexuality with a health professional than those with a cancer that commonly impacts sexuality, such as prostate, testicular, breast, or gynecologic cancer. However, it is not only cancers that affect sexual or reproductive sites of the body that impact sexuality, and discussion and information about sexuality is needed across all types of cancer.

Older People

There is evidence that some health professionals do not provide information or communicate about sexuality with their older patients, as they assume older people are asexual or are likely to be offended if the issue is raised. Older patients have been described as not "worrying about sexual contact so much," "over the sex," and "not as sexually active as a young group of people." This functioned to position sex as unimportant or less important for older individuals. While sexual functioning does decline with age and illness, there is consistent evidence that many older adults are sexually active and that sex remains an important aspect of well-being in later life. It should not be assumed that sexual health information and support is not relevant or needed by older people.

LGBTQI Patients and Partners

Sexual concerns of LGBTQI patients are less likely to be addressed than those of heterosexual and cisgender individuals (see Chapter 5). Healthcare professionals often assume patients are heterosexual and provide heteronormative information and advice. LGBTQI patients and their partners can experience this as homophobic and discriminatory. If sexual minority patients disclose their sexuality, the response of health professionals can range from accepting to ignoring or rejecting the disclosure. Some clinicians are reticent to discuss sexuality or provide relevant sexual information in response to disclosure. It has been suggested that this is because they lack knowledge and training regarding the sexual practices of sexual minorities and have concerns about appropriate use of language. Disclosure of sexual orientation in order to receive targeted information and support can be a focus of difficulty for LGBTQI individuals. Disclosure of sexual orientation to health professionals is associated with positive mental health outcomes and greater satisfaction with care. In contrast, nondisclosure has been associated with fear of mistreatment, privacy concerns, and uncertainty as to whether sexual orientation is important to medical care.

Culturally and Linguistically Diverse (CALD) People

Migrant people from diverse ethnic and cultural backgrounds may experience a number of barriers to receiving support in relation to cancer and sexuality. First, in some cultural contexts, topics related to sexuality are considered private and taboo, and therefore silenced. This in part may explain why people from CALD backgrounds often report low levels of need for information about sexuality. However, a reluctance to address sexual changes or access information may mean that concerns go unaddressed, leading to heightened distress and relational difficulty. Even when CALD people with cancer may like to address sexual concerns, low levels of spoken English can result in communication difficulties with healthcare professionals or a reluctance to voice needs in the presence of an interpreter. Written resources may also not be accessible for CALD people, particularly if they have poor written English literacy or low literacy in their own language. CALD people with cancer may also be migrating from contexts where the healthcare systems are vastly different from those in developed contexts. This can result in difficulties navigating the healthcare system, or not being aware of certain services or entitlements (e.g., psychological/psychosexual support) that are available to them. Box 2.8 provides accounts of overcoming barriers to communication from the perspective of patients[11] and healthcare professionals.[15]

Overcoming Barriers to Communication

Lack of knowledge, confidence, or comfort on the part of health professionals in discussing sexuality with cancer patients has led to the development of brief training programs and publication of practical strategies to facilitate communication with patients about sex in the context of cancer. However, the success of such strategies depends on health professionals being reflexive

> **Box 2.8 Overcoming Barriers to Communication**
>
> *Patients*
> Permission; culturally sensitive information and support (across gender, cultural background, sexual identity, age); prompts and checklists as to how to raise the issue
>
> "I had a checklist of questions from the cancer council booklet, so knew what to ask and what to expect. It really helped when I talked to my doctor." (Ann, 22, hematologic cancer)
>
> "My oncologist and I are quite OK discussing sex. She doesn't necessarily ask, but if I talk about it then she'll respond to the questions." (Maeve, 49, breast cancer)
>
> "I brought up the stuff around sexual function myself. My oncologist handled it really well. He was really, really good with all of that and very understanding about me being a gay man." (James, 56, prostate cancer)
>
> *Healthcare Professionals*
> Education/training; having sexuality on the agenda; clinical guidelines; resource availability; referral pathways
>
> "There's a good brochure on sex after treatment for prostate cancer. I will give them that and then talk about it at the next session, saying, 'Have you read that brochure? What do you think?'" (Andrea, doctor, urology)
>
> "In the inpatient setting, because privacy can be an issue, often I will try and go back a second time and see if I can catch them either alone, or just with their partner, and if possible do it then." (Cathy, psychologist, general oncology)
>
> "Putting it on the agenda for all health professionals is really important, because I think otherwise people assume that it's the counselor's business or the social worker's business or the nurse's business or someone else—and then we don't talk about it." (Maree, nurse, general oncology)
>
> "I suppose when it comes to raising sexuality issues what we normally say is our number-one rule is to assume nothing, so we ask everybody no matter what their age, their cultural background, their relationship status because from time to time we have had people raise questions that we might not otherwise have predicted." (Maria, psychologist, general)

in their practice, acknowledging their own limitations, and accepting the need for professional training or development. Having awareness of communication strategies to raise sexual concerns with cancer patients and their partners is the first step.

How to Communicate About Sex with Cancer Patients and their Partners

The BETTER model[14] was specifically developed as a tool to help oncology nurses include sexuality in their general patient assessments (Box 2.9). It can

> **Box 2.9 The BETTER Model of Sexual Communication in the Context of Cancer**
>
> **Bring** up the topic of sexuality with cancer patients and their partners.
>
> **Explain** you are concerned with quality-of-life issues, including sexuality and sexual well-being. You may not be able to address all concerns, but let patients and their partners know that they can raise problems or concerns with you.
>
> **Tell** patients that you will find appropriate information or support services to address their concerns.
>
> **Timing** for discussion of sexuality might not be right at the present time, but acknowledge that patients and partners can discuss sexual concerns at any time.
>
> **Educate** patients about impact of cancer treatments on sexuality and sexual well-being.
>
> **Record** your assessment of sexual concerns and any interventions in patients' medical records.

be used in conjunction with the PLISSIT model, as it provides a more detailed roadmap of how to raise the issue of sexuality with cancer patients and their partners. The first step is to bring up the topic of sexuality, creating the opportunity for patients to identify any concerns. Then explain that you are concerned with quality-of-life issues, which include sexual well-being, and let patients know that they can ask for information at any time. Investigate the severity of any sexual concerns and patients' ability to manage them. Tell patients that you will find appropriate information and resources to address sexual concerns. When you first meet patients or their partners, sexual well-being may not be high on their agenda, as the initial focus is usually on survival. However, identifying your willingness to discuss sexuality concerns will open the door for future communication. If appropriate, educate patients about the side effects of their cancer treatments on sexual well-being and intimate relationships by discussing or providing information. Determine patients' knowledge of sexual changes and their management as well as their understanding of what is happening and why, and what to anticipate. Education must include positive suggestions so that patients can maintain or resume intimate relationships. Lastly, record your assessment and interventions.

Other guidelines provide information about the specific language healthcare professionals might use in raising the issue of sexuality with cancer patients. The Brief Sexuality Related Communication for women with breast cancer, produced by Cancer Australia (2015), outlined in Box 2.10, is one example.

Ethical Dilemmas

Ethical dilemmas may arise when clinicians are asked to provide information and advice about sexual changes to patients who are under the age of sexual consent, or unmarried people from culturally diverse backgrounds where premarital sex is taboo. If the patient requires information about sexual

> **Box 2.10 The Brief Sexuality Related Communication for Women with Breast Cancer, Cancer Australia, 2015**
>
> **Support a woman to discuss her feelings.**
>
> Provide permission for a woman to discuss her sexual feelings and validate her experiences and concerns, noting that some women may feel guilt or embarrassment that they view their sexual well-being as a concern.
>
> *"Many women find that treatment for breast cancer changes their interest in sex and intimate relationships—this is more common than you may think, and it can have a big impact on your life."*
>
> **Support a woman to identify her sexual well-being concerns.**
>
> Support a woman to explore and prioritize her own sexual well-being concerns, noting that these may not be limited to physical symptoms.
>
> *"Many women experience side effects of treatments that impact relationships or sexual activities, such as loss of desire or pain. Do you feel that these or other symptoms are affecting your sex life or relationship? What do you (and your partner) find most concerning?"*
>
> **Support a woman to consider her expectations regarding her sexual well-being.**
>
> The changes to sexual well-being experienced may or may not be acceptable for a woman and her partner. Health professionals can encourage a woman and her partner to consider the ways in which they express sexuality and intimacy, and if they can explore alternative practices.
>
> *"Considering your symptoms, what would you (and your partner) consider an ideal outcome to be? How would you (and your partner) feel if you couldn't achieve this?"*
>
> **Provide information about what to expect.**
>
> Women should be aware that their sexual well-being concerns and priorities may change along the continuum of care associated with their treatment, their relationship with a partner, or their perception of themselves. Let the woman know that you are available to discuss sexual well-being at any stage and reinforce that her concerns are valid.
>
> *"You may not feel like thinking about or discussing your sexual well-being now, but you can always ask any questions you or your partner may have at any time in the future."*
>
> https://canceraustralia.gov.au/sites/default/files/publications/2013_sexual_wellbeing_online_resource.pdf

changes or concerns, it is the responsibility of the clinician to provide it or to refer the patient to an appropriate third party if intensive therapy is required.

Policies

All oncology treatment centers should include acknowledgment of the impact of cancer treatment on sexual well-being and fertility in policies that govern patient information and care. Such policies should include provision of information about sexual changes and infertility, and referral sources for those who need intensive therapy or intervention.

Teams and Supervision

All members of clinical teams should be provided with training and supervision in how to communicate about sexual concerns that occur in the context of cancer. It is recommended that there is at least one member of a team who has in-depth expertise in addressing sexual issues and who can deal with more complex cases and provide supervision for junior team members in appropriate ways of communicating about sex and sexuality.

Conclusion

Changes to sexuality can be experienced as one of the most difficult aspects of life following cancer. This can include changes to sexual functioning, body image, fertility, and gender identity. Such changes are multifaceted and linked with a range of negative physical and emotional outcomes for both people with cancer and their partners, as well as changes to roles and intimate relationships. There is evidence that people with cancer and their partners report the need for information and support to address sexual concerns after cancer from health professionals; however, such information provision is often inadequate or absent.

Healthcare professionals can play an important role in ameliorating concerns about sexual well-being after cancer by (1) giving permission for the discussion of sexual matters, (2) offering introductory information on sexual changes, and (3) making specific suggestions about renegotiating sex, following the PLISSIT model. Such patient education and support about the impact of cancer on sexual well-being should include information on the whole spectrum of sexual activities available for maintaining intimacy and sexual satisfaction, rather than focusing on coital sex. If information provision is not sufficient for an individual or couple, referral for intensive therapy may be appropriate.

References

1. Perz J, Ussher JM, Gilbert E. Feeling well and talking about sex: psycho-social predictors of sexual functioning after cancer. *BMC Cancer* 2014;14(1):228–247.
2. Schover LR, van Der Kaaij M, van Dorst E, et al. Sexual dysfunction and infertility as late effects of cancer treatment. *EJC Suppl* 2014;12:41–53.
3. Gilbert E, Ussher JM, Perz J. Sexuality after breast cancer: a review. *Maturitas* 2010;66:397–407.
4. Gilbert E, Ussher JM, Perz J. Sexuality after gynaecological cancer: a review of the material, intrapsychic, and discursive aspects of treatment on women's sexual well-being. *Maturitas* 2011;70(1):42–57.
5. Parton CM, Ussher JM, Perz J. Women's construction of embodiment and the abject sexual body after cancer. *Qual Health Res* 2016;26(4):490–503.
6. Jankowska M. Sexual functioning of testicular cancer survivors and their partners—a review of literature. *Rep Pract Oncol Radiother* 2012;17(1):54–62.
7. Rhoten BA. Head and neck cancer and sexuality: a review of the literature. *Cancer Nurs* 2016;39(4):313–320.

8. Traa MJ, De Vries J, Roukema JA, Den Oudsten BL. Sexual (dys)function and the quality of sexual life in patients with colorectal cancer: a systematic review. *Ann Oncol* 2012;23(1):19–27.

9. Ussher JM, Perz J, Kellett A, et al. Health-related quality of life, psychological distress, and sexual changes following prostate cancer: a comparison of gay and bisexual men with heterosexual men. *J Sex Med* 2016;13(3):425–434.

10. Ussher JM, Perz J, Gilbert E, et al. Renegotiating sex after cancer: resisting the coital imperative. *Cancer Nurs* 2013;36(6):454–462.

11. Gilbert E, Perz J, Ussher JM. Talking about sex with health professionals: the experience of people with cancer and their partners. *Eur J Cancer Care* 2016;25:280–293.

12. Perz J, Ussher JM, Australian Cancer and Sexuality Study Team. A randomised trial of a minimal intervention for sexual concerns after cancer: a comparison of self-help and professionally delivered modalities. *BMC Cancer* 2015;15(629):1–16.

13. Annon JS. PLISSIT therapy. In: Corsine RJ, editor. *Handbook of Innovative Psychotherapies*. New York: Wiley and Sons, 1981:629–639.

14. Mick J, Hughes M, Cohen M. Using the BETTER model to assess sexuality. *Clin J Oncol Nurs* 2004;8(1):84–86.

15. Ussher JM, Perz J, Gilbert E, et al. Talking about sex after cancer: a discourse analytic study of health care professional accounts of sexual communication with patients. *Psychol Health* 2013;28(12):1370–90.

16. Hawkins Y, Ussher JM, Gilbert E, et al. Changes in sexuality and intimacy after the diagnosis of cancer: the experience of partners in a sexual relationship with a person with cancer. *Cancer Nurs* 2009;34(4):271–280.

Further Reading

Benoot C, Saelaert M, Hannes K, Bilsen J. The sexual adjustment process of cancer patients and their partners: a qualitative evidence synthesis. *Arch Sex Behav* 2017;46(7):2059–2083. doi:10.1007/s10508-016-0868-2

A review of psychological interventions to address sexual changes after cancer

Cancer Council of New South Wales. Sexuality, intimacy and cancer. 2019. https://www.cancercouncil.com.au/wp-content/uploads/2014/05/UCPUBS1.pdf

Example of information that can be provided to patients experiencing sexual changes after cancer

Candy B, Jones L, Vickerstaff V, et al. Interventions for sexual dysfunction following treatments for cancer in women. *Cochrane Database Syst Rev* 2016;2(2):CD005540. doi:10.1002/14651858.CD005540.pub3

A review of interventions for women who experience sexual difficulties after cancer treatment

Carter J, Lacchetti C, Rowland JH. Interventions to address sexual problems in people with cancer: American Society of Clinical Oncology clinical practice guideline adaptation summary. *J Oncol Pract* 2018;14(3):173. doi:10.1200/JOP.2017.028134

Clinical guidelines on addressing sexual problems in people with cancer

Lipshultz LI, Pastuszak AW, Goldstein AT, et al. *Management of Sexual Dysfunction in Men and Women: An Interdisciplinary Approach*. New York: Springer, 2016.

A general text on sexual difficulties and how to manage them clinically

Chapter 3

Lesbian, Gay, Bisexual, and Transgender Issues

Karolina Lisy, Nick Hulbert-Williams, Jane M. Ussher, Alison Alpert, Charles Kamen, and Michael Jefford

Learning Objectives

After reading this chapter the clinician will be able to:

1. Understand the basic background of minority stress and discrimination faced by LGBT people
2. Recognize the unique issues that may be experienced by LGBT people with cancer and their partners
3. Inquire appropriately about sexual orientation and gender identity and use inclusive language
4. Be aware of available resources for LGBT people with cancer
5. Provide appropriate care for LGBT people with cancer

Background Evidence

Intention

This chapter will address some specific issues related to the sexual health, fertility, and relationships of lesbian, gay, bisexual, and transgender (LGBT) people with cancer and will discuss some general concepts regarding appropriate and respectful cancer care for LGBT patients. Many of the sexual health, relationship, and fertility issues discussed in other chapters in this book will also be relevant to LGBT people, for example the impacts of cancer treatment on fertility (see Chapter 1); however, the intention here is to focus on aspects of cancer and cancer care that affect LGBT people specifically.

Definitions and Scope

Though the focus of this chapter is people who identify as LGBT, we acknowledge that the term LGBT does not encompass the full spectrum of sexual orientations, gender identities, or sex characteristics that exist. Some of the more frequently used terms for diverse sexual orientations and gender identities (SOGI) are listed in Box 3.1.

> **Box 3.1 Sexual and Gender Identity Terms**
>
> *Sexual Identity Terms*
>
> **Asexual:** A sexual orientation generally characterized by not feeling sexual attraction toward others or having no desire for partnered sexuality
>
> **Bisexual:** A person whose primary sexual and affectional orientation is toward people of the same and other genders, or toward people regardless of their gender
>
> **Gay:** A sexual and affectional orientation toward people of the same gender. Typically used for men whose primary sexual and affectional orientation is toward other men
>
> **Heterosexual:** A person whose primary sexual and affectional orientation is toward people of the opposite gender
>
> **Homosexual:** A person whose primary sexual and affectional orientation is toward people of the same gender. The term "homosexual" is considered to be outdated as it was used historically to describe same-sex attraction as a mental disorder, and use of this term is not recommended
>
> **Lesbian:** A woman whose primary sexual and affectional orientation is toward other women
>
> **Pansexual:** A person who has sexual or affectional desire for people of all genders and sexes
>
> **Queer:** An inclusive term for people who identify as nonheterosexual, including but not limited to LGBT people. The term "queer" may have negative connotations for some LGBT people. It is not recommended that non-LGBT people use this term
>
> **Questioning:** A person who is unsure about or is exploring their sexual orientation and/or their gender identity
>
> *Gender Identity Terms*
>
> **Cisgender:** A person whose gender aligns with their sex at birth
>
> **Gender fluid:** A person whose gender identity is not fixed and who may move between genders
>
> **Genderqueer:** A person who doesn't identify with conventional binary gender identities
>
> **Nonbinary:** A person who does not identify as either male or female
>
> **Transgender:** A person whose gender identity differs from sex assigned at birth
>
> **Transgender man/transman/female-to-male (FTM):** A person assigned female sex at birth who identifies as male
>
> **Transgender woman/transwoman/male-to-female (MTF):** A person assigned male sex at birth who identifies as female

Though LGBT is a commonly used acronym to describe people who identify as sexually or gender diverse, other acronyms also exist, such as LGBTQ (Q = queer/questioning), LGBTI (I = intersex), and LGBTQIAP (A = asexual, P = pansexual). Longer acronyms may also be represented by LGBTQ+ to denote the other identities not explicitly included. We use the term LGBT in this chapter because the vast majority of research underpinning the text concerns people who identify as LGBT, with little reference to people from other SOGI groups. We also wish to distinguish between gender (a social construct) and sex (a set of biologic characteristics). Though gender identities are sometimes stated as including people who are intersex, we note that biologic sex characteristics do not fall within the social construct of gender. There may also be separate considerations for intersex people not covered in this chapter and not represented in the available evidence.

The LGBT Cancer Population

Because data regarding SOGI are not routinely collected in population surveys or censuses, or in cancer registries, exact numbers of LGBT people in the community and those affected by cancer are not known. Estimates of the numbers of LGBT people vary, although it is thought that between 3% and 12% of populations across countries identify as sexually or gender diverse. Considering that in 2018 there were an estimated 18.1 million new cancer diagnoses worldwide, it may be extrapolated that there were between 543,000 and 2,172,000 LGBT people diagnosed with cancer worldwide in the last year alone. These figures may indeed be conservative, as segments of the LGBT population have been reported to have elevated cancer risk factors such as smoking and obesity, and to experience higher rates of cancer.

Minority Stress

People who identify as LGBT may be at greater risk of inferior psychosocial outcomes following a cancer diagnosis compared with the general population. Minority stress theory proposes that external and intrinsic stressors that LGBT people experience lead to increased risk of psychological and mood disorders.[1] External stressors include discriminatory treatment, harassment, violence, and victimization, while internal or intrinsic stressors include concealment of LGBT identity, expectation of rejection, and hypervigilance. LGBT people are also more likely to experience stressful circumstances and life events, are more likely to be estranged from their families of origin, and, for older people, are less likely to have adult children who may participate in their care. For many LGBT people, worries about social isolation, vulnerability, and a future need for caregiving are prevalent. Indeed, elevated rates of depression, mood and anxiety disorders, suicidal ideation, and suicide attempt are observed in LGBT populations compared with heterosexual cisgender populations.[2] LGBT cancer populations have also been found to experience lower self-esteem and more relationship and social problems than heterosexual groups.[3] For example, in one US national survey, 10.1% of cancer survivors reported poor mental health–related quality of life, compared with only 5.9% of adults without a history of cancer.[4]

LGBT Rights

Progress toward legal and societal equality for LGBT people is being made in many countries; a significant example of this includes the recent recognition of same-sex marriage in much of the Western and developed world, including the United Kingdom, the United States, Australia, and New Zealand, as well as many countries throughout Western and Northern Europe, and

South America. However, the relatively recent decriminalization of homosexuality (mostly between men) and declassification of homosexuality as a mental illness warrants mention. Homosexuality was declassified by the American Psychiatric Association's *Diagnostic and Statistical Manual of Mental Disorders* (DSM) as a mental illness in 1973. Homosexual acts between men were decriminalized in the United Kingdom in 1967, in Canada in 1969, and across Australian states between 1973 and 1997; though legislation varies across the United States, homosexual acts between consenting adults have been legal nationwide only since 2003. India, the second most populous country in the world, decriminalized homosexuality in September 2018. At the time of writing, homosexuality remains a criminal offense in over 70 countries around the world. Cancer does not discriminate, and so how we care for cancer patients must be situationally contextualized. Depending on country of residence or origin, disclosure of sexual orientation and open discussion about nonheterosexual relationships will still be impossible for many.

LGBT Cancer Care

People who identify as LGBT may have unique needs and challenges in the context of their cancer experience and care. Research into the cancer needs of LGBT populations is gaining pace, with a rapidly evolving literature beginning to describe the experiences of LGBT people in the context of accessing and receiving care for their cancer. Evidence shows that collectively and individually, LGBT people have experienced, and continue to experience, discrimination when accessing cancer care; numerous studies have reported on negative experiences of LGBT people in the context of accessing cancer care.[5] Discrimination may be in the form of explicit abuse or rejection by healthcare professionals and refusal of healthcare, but also in lack of competent, relevant, and affirming care; lack of family or spousal recognition; lack of insurance coverage; and lack of representation in healthcare structures.

Recent data indicate that LGBT cancer survivors are less satisfied with the care they receive compared with heterosexual cancer survivors; they report being less likely to be included in decision-making and less likely to feel as though they are treated with dignity and respect by clinicians.[6] Regarding support groups, the literature also indicates that for LGBT people affected by cancer, including patients, caregivers, and their broader support networks, available support groups are often not appropriate or responsive to LGBT needs.[5]

Knowledge Gaps

Much of the current understanding of LGBT cancer experiences has arisen from investigations of gay and bisexual men with prostate cancer and lesbian and bisexual women with breast cancer, with scant literature addressing the needs of LGBT people with other cancer types. Furthermore, bisexual and transgender people remain further hidden within the LGBT literature, with few studies available that focus only on the experiences and outcomes of these groups. These are important gaps as we know that bisexual people face unique cancer-related issues and increased stigma, even within the LGBT community, and that transgender people are also most likely to experience discrimination and outright rejection when accessing healthcare.[7] It is also important to recognize that much of our research and knowledge of LGBT cancer experiences is based largely on Western, white LGBT people. We recognize that LGBT people in different ethnic and cultural groups may have intersecting needs that are underexplored and unknown.

Barriers to Best Care

One substantial barrier to quality cancer care for LGBT people is that clinicians may not have sufficient knowledge about LGBT health to provide appropriate care. LGBT health does not form a large part of current clinical curricula; as an example, US medical schools have a median of 5 hours of LGBT content, with some schools not providing any LGBT education at all. A recent survey of oncologists demonstrates that oncologists feel their knowledge is suboptimal, especially in regard to transgender health.[8]

Providers may also have their own biases when it comes to treating LGBT patients or feel insufficiently informed to talk to LGBT patients about their sexual health needs. One large US study demonstrated that healthcare providers, including physicians, mental health workers and nurses, exhibited implicit bias against gay men and lesbian women.[9] Suggestions for combating negative attitudes towards LGBT people include more positive experiences with LGBT patients and exposure to LGBT people, and greater education and inclusion of LGBT identities in training.

Presenting Problems

Usually, this title refers to medical diseases, illnesses, or predicaments for which patients seek assistance from providers. Here, what we refer to are clashes between LGBT people and medical structures that are often created with cisgender, heterosexual people in mind. In addition, we describe specific issues for LGBT patients during cancer treatment and survivorship. Presenting problems are summarized in Box 3.2.

Stigma and Discrimination

⚠ Previous experience of stigma and discrimination within the health care system may lead to mistrust or fear when accessing healthcare and may also lead to reduced access to essential healthcare services. This risk may be elevated for transgender people, more of whom report having experienced discriminatory treatment or outright rejection when accessing healthcare in the past. Patients may feel a heightened sense of alertness around new providers and may be unsure about how they will be treated or about the quality of care they may receive once they come out. Accessing care in religiously affiliated hospitals or services may be particularly stressful.

> **Box 3.2 Issues Complicating Cancer Care for LGBT People**
>
> - Healthcare providers often assume heterosexuality and cisgender identities.
> - Healthcare providers may not ask about SOGI and may not use their preferred name or pronouns.
> - Patient may or may not feel or be safe to discuss SOGI data.
> - Patients may have had previous negative healthcare experiences.
> - Resources available to support sexual health, fertility, and relationships reflect only heterosexual and cisgender identities and exclude LGBT experiences or concerns.
> - LGBT people are more likely to be estranged from their families of origin.
> - Older LGBT people are less likely to have adult children who may provide support and care.
> - Healthcare providers may lack knowledge and cultural competency to discuss specific LGBT issues with patients.
> - Additional stigma may be experienced by people with HPV-related cancers or for people who are living with HIV.

Heteronormativity

The term "heteronormativity" refers to the view that being heterosexual and cisgender is the norm or default orientation and gender identity, and that LGBT people who deviate from this norm are "other." Heteronormativity is often reflected in health systems through exclusive representation of heterosexual relationships in patient information, an emphasis on heterosexual sexual health, and a lack of LGBT inclusion in patient intake forms, to give a few examples.

⚠ Lack of LGBT representation may lead to LGBT people feeling "invisible" or unwelcome when accessing care. Gendered healthcare settings may be experienced as particularly uncomfortable for transgender or gender-diverse people—for example, a woman attending a men's health clinic or vice versa.

Assumptions of Cisgender and Heterosexual Identities

Heteronormativity may manifest in assumptions that patients are cisgender and/or heterosexual. Assumptions of cisgender heterosexual identity may be communicated by language choices that imply gender or sexual orientation—for example, assuming that a person is heterosexual and referring to their wife or husband, rather than asking if they have a partner. Language that assumes heterosexual or cisgender identities may put patients in the uncomfortable position of having to "come out," which may not feel safe, may cause distress, or may lead LGBT patients to lie about their SOGI, which may add to their psychological burden (see the section on minority stress earlier in the chapter[1]) and may lead to incomplete or inappropriate care.

Disclosure of SOGI

Knowledge of a person's SOGI is useful for enabling meaningful interactions between patients and providers and provision of tailored and appropriate care. For example, knowing a patient's SOGI can assist providers in making informed recommendations regarding fertility, sexual health, and tailored support services. Patients, however, may not feel or be safe disclosing their SOGI due to the possibility of discrimination, maleficence, or denials of care. Additionally, patients may wait for signals from their provider that it is safe to discuss SOGI data, or patients may feel that their SOGI may not be relevant to their care and may prefer to keep this information private. Nondisclosure may lead to inappropriate care or care that does not adequately address the needs of the LGBT person. Conversely, positive disclosure experiences have been shown to be associated with greater patient satisfaction with care.

Patient–Provider Interactions

Positive and effective verbal and nonverbal communication is important in establishing rapport and trust with LGBT patients.[10] This includes verbal and nonverbal displays of compassion, respect, and genuine interest in the patient. Conversely, language or behaviors that communicate stigmatization may decrease rapport and lead to decreased service usage. Negative reactions and behaviors can include changes in body language, eye contact, facial expressions, or tone of voice following disclosure. Stigmatizing verbal and nonverbal communication can occur in response to patients' gender presentation or expression, the presence of same-sex partners, or the presentation or expression of friends. Even neutral reactions to disclosure may be perceived negatively by LGBT patients.

Lack of LGBT-Specific Support Groups or Information Resources

LGBT patients with cancer often report that the care they receive does not meet their needs, leading to feelings of isolation, potentially through the entire trajectory of cancer diagnosis, treatment, and follow-up. LGBT people frequently report being dissatisfied with the level of information received regarding their sexual health and well-being during and following cancer treatment. This may be due to clinicians either not having the knowledge to answer their questions or not being comfortable discussing LGBT-specific issues. LGBT people further report a lack of relevant resources addressing their needs and a lack of LGBT-specific cancer support groups for both patients and partners or caregivers. General cancer support groups may not cater for the specific emotional, relationship, and sexual concerns of this population.

Nontraditional Relationships and Support Networks

LGBT people are less likely to have traditional support networks and more likely to have support provided by partners, former partners, and friendship networks; this is often referred to as the "family of choice" hypothesis and is far more common in LGBT communities than elsewhere. LGBT people may also reject social norms and conventions such as formal marriage and monogamy and maintain a variety of nontraditional relationships.

In the broader informal caregiving workforce, LGBT caregivers are significantly less likely to be a spouse or formal partner of the patient. Notably, LGBT people with cancer may be less likely than other demographic groups to want to involve their family and friends in their care and in decision-making. There are likely a myriad of potential causes for this, but one key theory is that this is done to protect significant others from the risk of discrimination and poor treatment in the traditionally heteronormative clinical care setting.

Increasingly, LGBT people, particularly in younger generations, feel able to live more openly with a same-gender partner, and to thus involve that partner in their healthcare. Research has highlighted some differences that may exist for LGBT caregivers: They are typically younger and more ethnically diverse and are more likely to report higher levels of financial strain associated with their caregiving role than their heterosexual counterparts.

Depression/Anxiety

⚠ For reasons described in the introduction to this chapter, the incidence of depression, anxiety, and suicidality is higher in LGBT people compared with the general population. For example, transgender patients have rates of suicide attempts that are nine times the national average. Discrimination or stigma due to SOGI can adversely affect a person's mental health, and the experience of cancer can exacerbate or trigger mental health issues. Marginalization related to LGBT identities and cancer may dovetail to worsen mental health. Given this, providers should be aware of LGBT patients' elevated risks for mental health issues and potential need for support services.

Stigma Related to Cancers Associated with Human Papillomavirus (HPV) and Human Immunodeficiency Virus (HIV)

HPV and HIV are sexually transmitted viruses that can affect any person who has been sexually active regardless of their SOGI. HIV does, however, disproportionately affect some segments of the LGBT population, specifically gay and bisexual men and transgender women.

HPV-associated cancers, such as head and neck, anal, cervical, and penile cancers, may be associated with greater stigma, distress, and feelings of self-blame or shame, given that these cancers can be associated with sexual activity. Patients with HPV-associated cancers may also have fears of passing HPV on to their partners. Having an HPV-associated cancer may be associated with adverse social and psychological consequences that leave people worried about disclosing their diagnosis to partners and worried about their sexual relationships. HPV vaccination is now widely recommended and should reduce the incidence of HPV-associated cancers in the future.

People living with HIV may similarly experience stigma regarding their serologic status. They are at a higher risk of some virus-related cancer types compared with people who are HIV negative. These risks are directly related to the burden of immunosuppression, commonly understood by measurement of the CD4 count. Overall, people infected with HIV are 1.69

times as likely than the general population to be diagnosed with any type of cancer.[11] Three cancers—Kaposi sarcoma, some subtypes of non-Hodgkin lymphoma, and cervical cancer—are known as acquired immunodeficiency syndrome (AIDS)-defining cancers because a diagnosis of one of these cancers in an HIV-positive person may indicate the onset of AIDS. Though increasing use and access to antiretroviral therapy have caused the incidence of cancer in HIV-infected people to decline, recent data show that the rates of AIDS-defining cancers and other virus-related cancers are still greater in people who are infected with HIV compared to the general population.[11] In terms of AIDS-defining cancers, people living with HIV are 498 times more likely to be diagnosed with Kaposi sarcoma, 12 times more likely to be diagnosed with AIDS-defining non-Hodgkin lymphoma, and, among women, 3 times more likely to be diagnosed with cervical cancer. People living with HIV are also 19 times more likely to be diagnosed with anal cancer, 3 times more likely to be diagnosed with liver cancer, and about 2 times as likely to be diagnosed with oropharyngeal cancer.[11] Oncologists must think closely about medication interactions for patients receiving antiretroviral therapy because a number of interactions have been noted between chemotherapy and antiretroviral drugs. These interactions may increase toxicity or decrease efficacy.

Clinical Management

General Recommendations

Ensure a Welcoming and Inclusive Environment
Small actions can go a long way to addressing the heteronormative healthcare environment. Environmental cues like the following can reduce stigma, reflect safety, and give a clear and consistent message of acceptance to LGBT service users:

- Display rainbow logos, provide staff with rainbow lanyards, and display posters and other materials showing same-sex couples and gender nonconforming individuals.
- Clearly post nondiscrimination policies in waiting rooms or common areas.
- Use inclusive and gender-neutral language on forms to allow for same-sex partners (i.e., "partner" or "spouse" instead of "husband/wife") and to distinguish between sex assigned at birth and gender (including space for preferred pronouns such as she/he, her/him, and them/they).

⚠ Seventy percent of transgender people have experienced harassment when using public bathrooms; therefore, provision of gender-neutral facilities (where feasible) is recommended. This can be either a single stall or unisex bathroom. If this is not possible, displaying posters or signs in bathrooms explaining gender diversity to other users may help transgender people feel more comfortable and protected when using the bathroom of their choice.

Avoid Making Assumptions About Sexual Orientation and Gender Identity

⚠ It is important not to make assumptions about a person's sexuality or gender and not to use language that may be alienating to an LGBT person:

- Avoid addressing women with the title "Mrs."
- Avoid using the terms "wife" or "husband" to ask about a patient's spouse or marital status.
- Ask nongendered questions like, "Who takes care of you?" "Who is supporting you?" or "Who else lives with you in the home?" to assess support systems without assuming heteronormative relationship structures. Do so without judgment. Done routinely as a way to get to know the person, questions may include names, age, occupations, and wellness of any partner(s) or dependents. The length or nature of any relationship may provide the clinician with an opportunity to affirm the importance of that partnership.

Facilitate Disclosure of SOGI

⚠ Healthcare providers need to be aware that disclosure of SOGI may cause stress and apprehension for an LGBT patient.

- Use neutral and inclusive language, such as "partner" or "spouse," until the patient indicates the gender of their partner. To ascertain the patient's marital or relationship status, ask "Do you have a partner?" and "Is your partner male or female?"
- Routinely ask every patient about their preferred name and pronouns. This can initiate a conversation about SOGI. Assess possibilities for including SOGI items as part of your clinic's intake process, preferably on forms or other nonverbal means of disclosure.
- Assure patients of the confidentiality of their information and tell them why it is relevant to their care.
- Respond respectfully and positively when a person discloses they are LGBT. But if a patient does not wish to disclose, respect this decision.
- Be aware of personal reactions to LGBT disclosure. Maintain a nonjudgmental and positive stance both to patients and their support partners. When breaches in communication occur, apologize and express your commitment to respecting the patient ("I apologize. I did not mean to be disrespectful").
- Be aware of the potential for heightened distress or mental health issues in LGBT patients. Empathize with any experiences of stigma or marginalization that patients may have experienced previously.

⚠ Disclosure of transgender status may be particularly stressful for a patient, and transgender people may also feel distress during procedures that require exposure of their bodies, particularly genital or chest areas.

- If a transgender person's recorded sex or identification indicates a sex other than their gender identity, making a note on their chart to communicate this to other clinicians may help prevent negative

reactions from clinicians who may not be aware that a person is transgender, and save the patient from having to identify to multiple clinicians. Informing other providers and staff of the patient's preferred pronouns will also reduce errors in language used to address a transgender patient.
- Avoid discussing a person's gender where it may be overheard by other patients or staff not involved in the patient's care to maintain the privacy of the patient.

Provide Patient-Centered Care and Involve Patients in Decision Making

LGBT people may have different concerns or needs related to their cancer, treatment, or supportive care due to their SOGI that must be considered by the clinician. Options must be thoroughly discussed and decisions made together with the patient. Treatment decisions may be influenced by SOGI, such as decisions between surgical treatments (e.g., deciding between breast-conserving surgery and mastectomy, and whether to have breast reconstruction) and hormonal therapies (e.g., those that may be gender affirming for transgender people). Gay or bisexual men may be more distressed than heterosexual men by sequelae of prostate cancer treatment such as penis shortening, loss of ejaculate, and loss of erection, and these concerns may have an impact on treatment decisions.

It is important to clearly discuss potential effects of treatment so patients can make informed choices regarding their care.

Include Partners and Families of Choice in Care

Recognition of nontraditional families and support networks is necessary to provide effective and sensitive care to LGBT patients. LGBT people in relationships may wish to be accompanied by their partner to appointments and to include their partner in discussions and in making decisions about their care. Some LGBT people may consider their most enduring and supportive relationships to be nonsexual partnerships, and care teams need to similarly acknowledge a patient's wish to involve a nonpartner family member or friend in their care and decision-making.

- Avoid making assumptions regarding the relationships of patients and their support people. Respectfully inquire about any support people present and listen to the patient's language when speaking about them.
- Refer to same-sex or same-gender partners or spouses using the patient's own terminology (e.g., partner, spouse, wife, or husband) rather than dismissing this person as a friend.
- Fully recognize same-sex or same-gender partners/spouses as integral members of the patient's support team. Treat them equally and afford them the same rights as heterosexual partners/spouses. This may include involving partners in appointments according to the wishes of the patient, treating partners with respect, recognizing partners as legitimate next of kin, and ensuring nondiscrimination in visitation policies.

- If a patient decides not to involve partners or family members in their care, respect this decision while being mindful that this may arise from fear or a desire to protect others.

Be Knowledgeable About LGBT-Specific Resources and Support Groups

Some general cancer and supportive care resources may not be relevant, appropriate, or of interest to LGBT people. LGBT people with cancer, and their partners or caregivers, may prefer to attend LGBT-specific support groups. Patients may feel disenfranchised when support and information resources are heteronormative and emphasize heterosexual sex and behaviors.

⚠ For example, the "pink culture" within breast cancer organizations and the focus on maintaining a feminine appearance after cancer treatment, in terms of support with makeup, hair, or wigs, may be alienating for some gender- and sexuality-diverse women.

Resources that include LGBT sexual health are slowly improving. While printed resources specific to LGBT people with cancer may be limited in some settings, there are a number of online information and support resources that may be suitable.

- Be prepared by knowing what information resources are available in print or online (see suggested resources in Box 3.3). Where available resources are limited in LGBT inclusivity or otherwise inadequate, verbally acknowledge this and offer to discuss any issues with the patient; a positive and interested manner will be well received.
- Investigate any LGBT-specific support groups in the local area, or appropriate online support groups, so you can offer LGBT patients options for support groups or peer support.

Case Study

Melanie is 39 and identifies as a lesbian. She has recently undergone external-beam radiotherapy and brachytherapy for cervical cancer and is experiencing sensations of vaginal dryness and lost libido, which she finds distressing. Attending a follow-up appointment with her radiation oncologist, Melanie explains how she is feeling and asks what she can do to address these issues. Her oncologist gives her some brief information on lubricants and tells her it is safe to resume having sex with her husband, and that any pain during intercourse should resolve on its own over time. Due to the oncologist's assumptions regarding her sexuality and hurried manner, Melanie feels too uncomfortable to say her partner is female and to ask for information that may be relevant to her. She leaves the appointment unsure of what she should do and unwilling to raise the subject again.

Support for the Partner

Same-sex or same-gender partners, and other people who are supporting LGBT people living with or beyond cancer, will require their own support to cope with the cancer experience, any relationship changes, or new roles as

Box 3.3 International Examples of Information Resources for LGBT People Living With and After Cancer

General Information for LGBT People and Cancer

Cancer Council (Australia) information about cancer support for LGBT people with cancer: https://www.cancercouncil.com.au/lesbian-gay-bi-sexual-transgender-and-intersex-communities-and-cancer-support/

CancerCare (United States) information resources for LGBT people with cancer: https://www.cancercare.org/tagged/lgbt

National LGBT Cancer Network (United States) information resources: https://cancer-network.org/cancer-information/

National LGBT Cancer Project (United States) LGBT cancer survivors support organization with information and survivor stories: https://lgbtcancer.org/

Cancer's Margins, a LGBT2Q Arts and Community–based project including digital patient stories (Canada): https://www.lgbtcancer.ca/the-cancers-margins-study-and-our-digital-stories/

Resources for Gay and Bisexual Men with Prostate Cancer

Prostate Cancer Foundation Australia suite of information booklets for gay and bisexual men with prostate cancer: http://www.prostate.org.au/awareness/for-recently-diagnosed-men-and-their-families/gay-and-bisexual-men/download-information/

Prostate Cancer UK information for gay and bisexual men with prostate cancer: https://prostatecanceruk.org/prostate-information/living-with-prostate-cancer/gay-and-bisexual-men

LGBT Walnut is a support group for LGBT people affected by prostate cancer: http://www.lgbt-walnut.org.uk/

Online support groups for men with prostate cancer, including a dedicated group for gay men: https://malecare.org/

Prostate Cancer Canada resource: http://www.prostatecancer.ca/Prostate-Cancer/Facing-Prostate-Cancer/Gay-and-Bisexual-Men-Prostate-Cancer

Resources for Adolescent and Young Adult LGBT People with Cancer

Peter MacCallum Cancer Centre and ONTrac at Peter Mac Adolescent and Young Adult (AYA) Cancer Service (Australia) information booklet: https://www.petermac.org/beingokbeingyou

Resources for Transgender and Gender-Diverse People with Cancer

National LGBT Cancer Network (United States) information resources specific for transgender and gender-diverse people with cancer: https://cancer-network.org/cancer-information/transgendergender-nonconforming-people-and-cancer/

a caregiver. Acknowledging and addressing these difficulties in partners and social networks is important not just for their own sake, but also because of the dyadic nature of distress: Increased psychological distress in partners also increases the likelihood of psychological distress experienced by the patient.

⚠ In just the same way that LGBT people with cancer may feel that general support groups are not applicable to their needs, same-sex partners and support systems may also feel uncomfortable attending general support groups for partners of people with cancer. Furthermore, support groups are often gender-biased and specifically tailored for heterosexual partners (e.g., "Supporting Blokes" for male partners of women with breast cancer).

Sexual Health

Sexual well-being may be impacted by the psychological burden of receiving a cancer diagnosis and also by treatment side effects such as reductions in sexual desire and satisfaction; pain during sex; erectile and ejaculation changes; changes in penis size; vaginal dryness, tightness, and narrowing; and incontinence during sex. In fact, for some people, sexual changes are the most distressing long-term effect of cancer. This is not limited to sex-related cancers but to all cancers and treatments that affect body structures and sexual functioning, as well as body image, fatigue, relationships, and fertility. All of these contribute to changes in a person's view of themselves as a sexual being. These changes can also have a negative impact on gender identity and sexual identity and can be a cause of psychological distress.

⚠ LGBT people's concerns related to sexual function and rehabilitation may not be the same as those of people who engage exclusively in heterosexual sex. For example, the impact of treatment on the sexual health and rehabilitation needs of a lesbian who does not participate in coital sex may not be the same as the impact for a heterosexual woman; another example may be the impact of surgery for colorectal cancer on a patient's ability to engage in anal sex. Given that most written patient information is focused on heterosexual and cisgender people, patients may not see themselves reflected in it.

Clinician should not make assumptions about a patient's sexual behavior. If clinicians assume that patients have heterosexual and cisgender identities, they may provide patients with irrelevant information that may be perceived as heterosexist or cisgenderist.

⚠ It is important not to assume the kind of sexual behaviors a person engages in, due to their sexual orientation or gender identity or expression. When asking about sexual behavior and activity, clinicians should be aware that there is substantial diversity in behavior, and gender identity is separate from sexual orientation and behavior. For example, a woman who identifies as a lesbian may still have sex with men. Someone who identifies as bisexual may currently be in a monogamous relationship with a partner of the same or opposite sex. A man who identifies as heterosexual may be married to a woman, but also have sex with men. A transgender person may identify as heterosexual, or as gay, lesbian, or queer.

- Be willing and open when discussing patients' sexual concerns.
- If you need knowledge about the patient's past or current sexual activity to provide care, use gender-neutral and inclusive questions and terms. Be nonjudgmental. Let patients know why they are being asked these questions and assure them that any discussions will remain confidential. Suggestions for asking about sexual activity include asking if the patient has sex with women, men, or both, and then what type of sex that person has (Box 3.4). Practice and become comfortable asking questions about sexual behavior.
- Avoid making assumptions about the sexual activities that LGBT people engage in based on their sexual orientation or gender expression. Instead, ask with sensitivity and respect about sexual behavior.

Box 3.4 Asking Questions About Sexual Behavior

Do not assume that a person is heterosexual. Ask the patient if they have a partner and about their current sexual activities. Give permission to describe behaviors and normalize these behaviors in an LGBT setting.

Some examples of how to ask about single or multiple partners and sexual activity:

'Are you currently sexually active?'

'Do you have a current sexual partner or partners?"

'Do you have sex with men, or women, or both men and women?'

'What types of partners have you been sexually active with over the last [insert clinically relevant length of time]: men, or women, or both men and women?"

'When you have sex, what type of sex do you have? Insertive anal (top), receptive anal (bottom), or both (versatile)? Oral? Vaginal? Any other types?'

Following treatment for cancer, changes to a person's sexual feelings and functioning may have occurred. Ask about these and what impact these may have on their well-being, sexual activity, and relationship(s). Ask patients about their goals for sexual rehabilitation and establish what matters to them. If the patient has a partner, ask about the couple's style of communication about these changes, and encourage communication within the couple. Ask what efforts have been attempted thus far to improve intimacy and sexual function. What works and what doesn't work?

- Be mindful of the diversity of sexual relationships that patients may have. These may include monogamous partners, multiple partners, open relationships, or casual partners/encounters.
- Seek knowledge of sexual issues and concerns that may affect LGBT patients in order to provide adequate care. Where your knowledge is lacking, displaying a positive and interested manner in response to sexual health needs or questions, and efforts to seek out information, will be well received.

Understanding the Sexual Needs of Gender- and Sexuality-Diverse Women

There is limited research on the sexual concerns of gender- and sexuality-diverse women following cancer; the focus has been on the experiences of lesbians with breast cancer. There is some evidence that lesbians experience psychological distress associated with greater social and relationship difficulties and greater disruption in sexual activity and desire in comparison to heterosexual women.[12] Conversely, other studies suggest that lesbians with cancer report lower levels of sexual concern and less disruption in sexual activity, as well as less concern about their appearance, than heterosexual women. Lesbians with breast cancer have also described themselves as "better off" than heterosexual women due to high levels of partner empathy and reduced focus on bodily appearance within their relationship. Cancer may have a different impact depending on age, with younger lesbian, bisexual, and queer women more concerned about changes to appearance and impact on future relationships. Older women may be more able to negotiate sexual changes, particularly if they are in an ongoing relationship.

Case Studies

Zoi is 28 and identifies as a bisexual. She has recently been diagnosed with and treated for breast cancer. She is highly distressed about the scarring on her breast following a lumpectomy and the impact of hormonal treatment on vaginal dryness and body weight. She feels as if she is going into menopause and is "old before my time." Zoi avoids any form of sexual relationship, as she doesn't want to expose her "deformed" body. She feels alienated from the queer community focus on the "body beautiful, and being sexy." She feels neither.

Helen is 55, identifies as a lesbian, and has been with her partner Maggie for 20 years. Maggie tells her she is still beautiful, and they have maintained intimacy in their relationship throughout the cancer treatment. After recovery from a double mastectomy, Helen decided to have a flower garland tattooed on her chest, which she loves. She had already gone through menopause so hadn't noticed the impact of hormonal treatment on her sexual well-being. Tiredness was the worst problem.

Understanding the Sexual Needs of Gay and Bisexual Men

There is consistent evidence that gay and bisexual men are more distressed by changes in sexual functioning and suffer from lower self-esteem and poorer self-image as a result of sexual changes associated with cancer and cancer treatment compared with heterosexual men.[3] However, gay and bisexual men are more likely to explore sexual rehabilitation following cancer and cancer treatment and to access support online or from a health professional.[13] Postcancer sexual changes may negatively impact other areas of well-being such as mental and emotional health, gay identity, social well-being and relationships, and overall quality of life.

⚠️ It is important for clinicians to understand the sexual behavior of gay and bisexual men so they can provide information and advice, and also to be comfortable and open with patients when discussing their sexual health. Some of the common concerns experienced by gay men following cancer treatment, and their impact on the patient, are as follows:

- Erectile dysfunction as a result of cancer treatment may be more bothersome in men who engage in anal sex as the insertive partner compared with heterosexual men. As a firmer erection is required for anal penetration compared with vaginal penetration, loss of erectile function may impede or inhibit anal sex following treatment.
- Erectile dysfunction may cause distress when engaging in other sexual activities, or for men who are the receptive partner, as a lack of erection can be interpreted as lack of arousal or interest.
- Prostatectomy will likely affect the sensation of anal sex for the receptive partner, and in some men may result in loss of pleasure.
- Body image issues may be worse for gay men who might compare their bodies and sexual functioning with that of their partner(s), making them feel inferior. This may be especially true regarding reduction in penis size following prostatectomy or radiation, and is posited as worse than the experience of heterosexual men, leading to a sense of inadequacy and body shame.
- Gay and bisexual men are more likely to have casual sexual partners, or multiple partners, which alters the context within which they have to renegotiate sex after cancer. Diminished sexual function due to cancer treatment may reduce the confidence of unpartnered men to approach potential partners.
- Gay men may be more bothered by lack of ejaculation, which may be experienced as diminished pleasure of orgasm and loss of visible evidence of sexual enjoyment with partners. This may lead to loss of confidence or feelings that partners are disappointed.
- Climacturia and urinary incontinence may lead to men avoiding sex with new, casual, or long-term partners. Men may feel awkward discussing their incontinence with partners.
- For partnered men, disruptions to sexual activity may lead to their partner exploring new sexual relationships outside of the couple or seeking an open relationship.

Overall, the sexual changes that gay and bisexual men might experience following cancer treatment cause substantial distress and loss of self-esteem, sense of self, and identity, and some men may experience regret about their treatment decisions once faced with these challenges. Compounding these issues are the barriers men face in seeking help, including not disclosing sexual orientation and lack of knowledge by healthcare providers about these issues.

Case Studies

Mark, age 49, described his gay identity as going through a "crisis" following prostate cancer. Sexual prowess was a fundamental part of his identity as a gay man, and he now felt inadequate and unattractive. His large penis had been a "calling card" and was "now gone." With a partial erection, he could no longer be the active partner in anal sex, and he didn't want to be the receptive partner: "It doesn't appeal to me at all." He no longer walked around naked in the gay sauna because he was embarrassed about his "small dick." He also avoided casual sex, where the absence of semen would have to be explained: "It would be too hard to kind of disclose or to pick up somebody and say, 'Well, nothing is going to happen on my part, you know . . . I can't cum.'" He said he felt he had been forcibly retired from the "gay human race."

David, 65, identified as a bisexual man but primarily had sex with men. He had explored a range of methods of sexual rehabilitation after prostate cancer. Cock rings and a vacuum pump had a limited effect, and taking sildenafil (Viagra) gave him a headache. Penile injections were the most effective, allowing him to have sex for prolonged periods, as long as the receptive partner "can take it." This made him feel "young" and attractive with "a lot of the younger guys attracted to me." He had also learned how to do sensual massage and to focus on sexual pleasure that didn't involve an erection. He said his sex life was better than ever.

Fertility

Many cancer treatments affect the fertility of patients. Some clinicians may assume that persons who are gay, lesbian, bisexual, or transgender will not be interested in having children. Such assumptions may lead to skipping critical discussions regarding the impacts of treatment on fertility and discussion about options for fertility preservation prior to treatment.

The impacts of cancer treatment on fertility, and guidance on fertility-preservation options, have been discussed elsewhere in this volume (see Chapter 1). For younger people with cancer who identify as LGBT, the consequences of cancer treatment on fertility are no different than for people who are cisgender and heterosexual. However, LGBT people have reported dissatisfaction with the amount and quality of information they received about fertility from clinicians, with some patients not being told about impacts on fertility until after treatment is completed. LGBT patients also have less available online information regarding their fertility than heterosexual and cisgender people.

As with the general population, attitudes to having children vary among people who are LGBT. Some may not want to have children or may place less importance on having biologic children, or may be open or even expect that they will have children in other ways, such as adoption, fostering, surrogacy, or egg or sperm donation. However, with evolving reproductive technologies, increased societal acceptance, and improved legal rights, LGBT people increasingly report a desire to experience biologic parenthood, and it is likely that more LGBT people will want biologic children in the future.

It is essential not to make assumptions about a person's desire to have biologic children based on their sexual orientation, gender identity, appearance, or gender expression. To help them make treatment decisions, all patients of reproductive age, regardless of sexual orientation or gender identity, must be given complete information about any potential changes to fertility, including fertility-preservation options (where possible) and fertility counseling. This information must be provided before treatment starts.

Fertility for transgender people with cancer may present additional considerations depending on whether or not the patient has had any prior fertility-preservation or gender-affirming procedures. Transwomen may have had prior semen cryopreservation, and transmen may have had prior egg or embryo cryopreservation. Ovarian preservation and testicular tissue preservation are also emerging techniques. Gender-affirming procedures may include surgical removal of the ovaries or testicles, or hormonal therapies that adversely affect fertility. Knowledge of a transgender patient's history is essential in providing quality care regarding fertility.

Clinicians must be aware of the fertility options relevant to LGBT patients. These include donor sperm insemination, in vitro fertilization, and egg donation and gestational surrogacy. Some partners may want to use in vitro fertilization during which one partner's eggs are inseminated and carried in the uterus of the other partner (Box 3.5).

Professional Issues and Service Implementation

Provide LGBT Cultural Competency Training for Staff

There is a clear need for LGBT cultural competency training for staff, including healthcare providers and also administrative staff who have patient contact. Such training should focus on the specific needs of LGBT people with cancer as well as language used in clinical communication. There is published literature (for example,[14]) that can be used to inform this. In order to equip our health care system for equality sustainability, this training cannot just be limited to in-workplace training; we need to ensure that appropriate equality and diversity content is included in training curricula for healthcare professionals. We would advocate that this training be provided in a way that gives credibility to the voices of LGBT people, so it may be helpful for at least part of it to be delivered by someone who is LGBT themselves.

> **Box 3.5 Checklist for Best Clinical Care of LGBT Cancer Patients**
>
> - Use environment cues to communicate that your facility is an inclusive and save clinical setting to LGBT patients.
> - Avoid making assumptions about the sexual orientation, sexual behavior, or gender identity of patients and partners.
> - Facilitate positive disclosure of SOGI. Ask about preferred pronouns and relationship status.
> - Include same-sex/same-gender partners and families of choice in care, if desired by the patient.
> - Provide nonjudgmental, competent, and patient-centred care.
> - Be open and willing to ask about and discuss the sexual concerns and needs of LGBT patients.
> - Be knowledgeable about LGBT-specific resources and support groups.

Establish Processes for Sensitive SOGI Disclosure

Healthcare Services may consider including questions on SOGI alongside the other demographic information collected at assessment. This information is usually kept on the patient's medical record for all care providers to see, thus limiting the stress involved in multiple disclosures, particularly at the already stressful points of clinical transition, for example into palliative care. Often this kind of information is collected verbally by an administrator when a patient checks in to the clinic, and this may not be an appropriate format. As services increasingly move towards the use of electronic devices to collect patient information, these methods could be used to collect this crucial patient information in a sensitive and private way. Where technology is limited, a simple paper-based demographic information sheet would suffice.

Ensure Clear Antidiscrimination Policies

Services must have clear and relevant diversity and LGBT antidiscrimination policies. These (1) act as a tool to enforce training and development; (2) provide a clear message to LGBT patients about the kinds of care they can expect to receive; and (3) provide a transparent method by which noncompliance becomes known and acted on. This stance may be communicated to patients by posting antidiscrimination policies in patient areas such as waiting rooms.

Facilitate LGBT Advocacy

Antidiscrimination policies may facilitate and support staff to act as champions for LGBT rights, to call attention to situations where a lack of diversity or inclusivity arises, or to intervene in situations where they witness discrimination. This may include discussion of hospital policies, the design of and language used on patient intake forms, and the choice of information materials or posters on display in common areas, to provide a few examples. Staff should feel safe and able to do this without fear of discrimination themselves.

Increase Access to LGBT-Specific Support Groups and Information Resources

We would encourage any organisation that provides support groups for cancer patients, partners, or caregivers to consider running separate groups for those who identify as LGBT. We further suggest that organisations review their current patient-facing resources for inclusivity and take steps to address any lack of diversity that may be found.

References

1. Meyer IH. Prejudice, social stress, and mental health in lesbian, gay, and bisexual populations: conceptual issues and research evidence. *Psychol Bull* 2003;129(5):674–697.

2. Institute of Medicine. *The Health of Lesbian, Gay, Bisexual, and Transgender People: Building a Foundation for Better Understanding.* Washington, DC: Institute of Medicine, 2011.

3. Ussher JM, Perz J, Kellett A, et al. Health-related quality of life, psychological distress, and sexual changes following prostate cancer: a comparison of gay and bisexual men with heterosexual men. *J Sex Med* 2016;13(3):425–434.

4. Weaver KE, Forsythe LP, Reeve BB, et al. Mental and physical health-related quality of life among U.S. cancer survivors: population estimates from the 2010 National Health Interview Survey. *Cancer Epidemiol Biomarkers Prev* 2012;21(11):2108–2117.

5. Lisy K, Peters MDJ, Schofield P, Jefford M. Experiences and unmet needs of lesbian, gay, and bisexual people with cancer care: a systematic review and meta-synthesis. *Psychooncol* 2018;27(6):1480–1489.

6. Hulbert-Williams NJ, Plumpton CO, Flowers P, et al. The cancer care experiences of gay, lesbian and bisexual patients: a secondary analysis of data from the UK Cancer Patient Experience Survey. *Eur J Cancer Care* 2017;26(4). doi:10.1111/ecc.12670

7. James SE, Herman JL, Rankin S, et al. *The Report of the 2015 U.S. Transgender Survey.* Washington, DC: National Center for Transgender Equality, 2016.

8. Schabath MB, Blackburn CA, Sutter ME, et al. National survey of oncologists at National Cancer Institute–designated comprehensive cancer centers: attitudes, knowledge, and practice behaviors about LGBTQ patients with cancer. *J Clin Oncol* 2019;37(7):547–558.

9. Sabin JA, Riskind RG, Nosek BA. Health care providers' implicit and explicit attitudes toward lesbian women and gay men. *Am J Public Health* 2015;105(9):1831–1841.

10. Alpert AB, Cichoski-Kelly EM, Fox AD. What lesbian, gay, bisexual, transgender, queer, and intersex patients say doctors should know and do: a qualitative study. *J Homosex* 2017;64(10):1368–1389.

11. Hernández-Ramírez RU, Shiels MS, Dubrow R, Engels EA. Cancer risk in HIV-infected people in the USA from 1996 to 2012: a population-based, registry-linkage study. *Lancet HIV* 2017;4(11):e495–e504.

12. Kamen C, Mustian KM, Jabson JM, Boehmer U. Minority stress, psychosocial resources, and psychological distress among sexual minority breast cancer survivors. *Health Psychol* 2017;36(6):529–537.

13. Ussher JM, Perz J, Rose D, et al. Sexual rehabilitation after prostate cancer through assistive aids: a comparison of gay/bisexual and heterosexual men. *J Sex Res* 2019;56(7):854–869.
14. Banerjee SC, Staley JM, Alexander K, et al. Encouraging patients to disclose their lesbian, gay, bisexual, or transgender (LGBT) status: oncology health care providers' perspectives. *Transl Behav Med* 2018. doi:10.1093/tbm/iby105

Further Reading

Lisy K, Peters MDJ, Schofield P, Jefford M. Experiences and unmet needs of lesbian, gay, and bisexual people with cancer care: a systematic review and meta-synthesis. *Psychooncol* 2018;27(6):1480–1489.

Qualitative systematic review describing the experiences of lesbian, gay, and bisexual people with cancer care and interactions with healthcare professionals.

Meyer IH. Prejudice, social stress, and mental health in lesbian, gay, and bisexual populations: conceptual issues and research evidence. *Psychol Bull* 2003;129:674–697.

Seminal paper describing minority stress theory.

Quinn GP, Sanchez JA, Sutton SK, et al. Cancer and lesbian, gay, bisexual, transgender/transsexual, and queer/questioning (LGBTQ) populations. *CA Cancer J Clin* 2015;65:384–400.

A thorough overview of seven cancers that disproportionately affect LGBT people, psychosocial issues for LGBT people with cancer, and clinical implications and strategies to improve care.

Schabath MB, Blackburn CA, Sutter ME, et al. National survey of oncologists at National Cancer Institute–designated comprehensive cancer centers: attitudes, knowledge, and practice behaviors about LGBTQ patients with cancer. *J Clin Oncol* 2019;37:547–558.

A national survey of US oncologists regarding attitudes and knowledge about LGBT people with cancer.

Chapter 4

Adolescents and Young Adults

Catherine Benedict, Zeba Ahmad, Vicky Lehmann, and Jennifer S. Ford

Learning Objectives

After reading this chapter the clinician will be able to:

1. Identify adolescents and young adults at risk for reduced sexual and/or reproductive health after cancer
2. Understand how cancer impacts sexuality and fertility directly and indirectly, including through treatment side effects, changes in body image or sense of self, interpersonal and relationship difficulties, and quality-of-life concerns
3. Understand the relevance of patient age and stage of development in relation to the impact of cancer and its treatment on sexual health and fertility
4. Discuss sexual dysfunction and reduced fertility with adolescent and young adult survivors and advise them on safe sexual practices, sexual recovery treatments to maintain health and intimacy, fertility preservation, and family-building options after cancer
5. Consider specific issues relevant to certain patient populations, including gender and sexual minorities and underage patients

Background Evidence

Adolescents and young adults (AYA) represent a unique patient population with a number of age-specific care needs that should be understood and attended to as a part of comprehensive cancer care.[1] The age range for defining AYA patient groups varies somewhat throughout the world but is most commonly either 15- to 29-year-olds or 15- to 39-year-olds. Nevertheless, many of the issues unique to AYA patients and survivors are consistent. Survival rates are generally high in AYA cancers, and many patients will face late and long-term side effects of treatment that impair quality of life.

The effects of cancer and its treatment on sexual functioning and fertility are common and are ranked as among the most distressing survivorship issues faced by this age group. Difficulties associated with sexuality, body image, and intimacy, facing infertility risk, and coping with loss of fertility are all relevant issues for patients across disease and treatment groups. Further, when cancer occurs during this age range, its sequelae can disrupt key developmental tasks and can have long-lasting effects on areas of life connected to and affected by sexual and reproductive health problems.

The broad effects of cancer during the AYA age range include disruption to and difficulties with dating, psychosexual maturation, establishing committed relationships, building intimacy with a romantic partner, understanding reproductive potential, and planning future family building. AYAs affected by cancer often must learn to adjust to a "new normal" in survivorship as they face ongoing late/long-term effects of treatment, such as sexual dysfunction or infertility, and/or altered expectations for achieving important life goals related to the pursuit of parenthood and building a family. These age-specific difficulties must be recognized and addressed as a part of cancer care with respect to patients' health status, developmental age, sexual maturity, and interest in and preferences for support.

Prevalence Data

Sexual dysfunction occurs in almost half of all AYA survivors and as many as one third of AYA survivors of childhood cancer, with estimates suggesting higher prevalence among females.[2,3] Rates of treatment-associated infertility vary widely (10% to 60%), depending on a number of factors such as age, reproductive health prior to cancer, and the toxicity of treatments. Clinical practice guidelines stipulate that addressing both sexual health and fertility should be essential components of AYA cancer care.[4]

Diverse Needs

Compared to pediatric and older adult patients, addressing the sexual and reproductive health needs of AYAs should be specific to this age group. At the same time, AYAs are also a diverse group, and supportive care services should be targeted and tailored to meet individual needs and preferences. Support needs often vary depending on where patients are in their cancer journey. Presenting problems change as patients move from active treatment to posttreatment survivorship, and by treatment-specific late-effect profiles. Patients on long-term maintenance or endocrine therapy (such as tamoxifen for breast cancer survivors) may also have concerns associated with ongoing treatment-related issues.

Childhood Cancer Survivors

Survivors of childhood cancer who were diagnosed at younger than age 15 and who have aged into the AYA age range have their own unique experiences and needs compared to those diagnosed during their AYA years. The long-term physical and psychosocial effects of experiencing cancer at a young age require special consideration. Practical and psychological factors may differ from patients diagnosed as AYAs, such as the involvement of parents in treatment and increased dependence on parents for navigating healthcare access. Sexual and reproductive health outcomes and supportive care needs may be similar, however, and clinicians may need to address such issues as a part of caring for childhood cancer survivors to ensure they are connected to the support and services they need.

Disruption of Development

A key aspect of sexual health for AYA survivors is the disruption of developmental activities related to psychosexual maturation. Treatment may cause significant disruption to the normal activities of adolescence and young adulthood related to exploring sexual identity, experimenting with sexual activities, and developing sexual relationships and intimacy with romantic partners. In addition to the direct effects of treatment, surviving cancer in young adulthood is associated with a disconnection from peers and potential feelings of social isolation, fear of dating, and less interest in sexual activity compared to same-age peers. Overall, AYA survivors have better physical functioning related to sexuality compared to those diagnosed as older adults, but AYAs report greater unmet needs related to sexual problems and concerns.

Risk-Taking Behaviors

AYA survivors of childhood cancer have been shown to exhibit increased risk-taking behaviors, including risky sexual behaviors. Childhood cancer survivors are less likely to use contraception and are at increased risk of contracting sexually transmitted infections. Poor psychological health among adolescent survivors of childhood cancer has been associated with early age sexual encounters and increased risk of unprotected sex, multiple lifetime sexual partners, and increased alcohol consumption and substance use.

Female Fertility Concerns

Concerns about fertility and future family building rank for many AYAs as one of the most distressing survivorship issues after a cancer diagnosis. For young women in particular, the prospect of infertility as a result of treatment causes immediate distress, and concerns persist well into survivorship, at times causing clinically significant depressive or anxiety symptoms and quality-of-life deficits. For others, fertility concerns arise later in life when survivors are ready for parenthood and want to start building their family, at which time they may realize that having a biologically related child is no longer possible. Alternatively, AYAs may assume they will be able to pursue family building using reproductive medicine, such as in vitro fertilization (IVF), or adoption, but come to realize that these options are much more complicated and challenging than anticipated. Thus, fertility-related distress may be a constant struggle for AYA survivors or occur more acutely at the time of family-building pursuits.

Male Fertility Concerns

Young men have reported lower distress in response to treatment-related infertility risks at the time of the cancer experience compared to women. However, evidence suggests men often report increased distress when pursuing family building later in life. A number of factors may be distressing for men, including sadness and regret if they are unable to have a biologically related child and being unable to pass on their genes to offspring, or feeling guilty if their female partner must undergo medical procedures such as IVF to become pregnant using their frozen sperm.

Gaps in Care

Patients are often not fully informed about the sexual side effects and infertility risks associated with treatment as a standard part of care, and as a result they are typically unprepared for the challenges they experience. Although many patients and survivors wish to discuss these issues with healthcare providers, barriers to having such discussions include patients' discomfort with the topics, providers' lack of knowledge and training, lack of time during clinic visits, and the presence of accompanying parents or partners who may overtly or inadvertently prevent discussions of sensitive or embarrassing topics. Compared to older adults, AYAs have reported higher levels of sexual symptoms and more unmet needs related to sexual dysfunction after cancer treatment. Likewise, fertility counseling is inconsistent across clinics at the time of diagnosis and even more intermittent regarding follow-up fertility care after treatment is completed.

Evidence-based structured interviews for healthcare providers to discuss sexual and reproductive health with AYAs have yet to be established, but a discussion guide based on the available research is provided in Table 4.1.

Clinical Practice Guidelines

Guidelines state that discussions about sexual side effects and referral for support should occur during the course of treatment for cancer patients and survivors of all ages. For AYAs in particular, guidelines stipulate that all patients of reproductive age should be counseled about infertility risks associated with treatment and made aware of fertility-preservation options when appropriate and available. Fertility counseling and fertility-preservation options are increasingly recognized and being offered as a standard part of care for AYAs. However, there are still notable gaps in care, and AYAs report high rates of unmet informational and supportive care needs related to sexual health and fertility concerns. Follow-up care for sexual dysfunction and fertility in survivorship is often missing or inadequate, despite consistent reports that AYAs want such services to be provided.

Addressing the medical and psychosocial difficulties associated with sexual and reproductive health problems across the continuum of cancer care is critical as patients and survivors have evolving questions, concerns, and needs. Providing support as AYAs move through diagnosis and treatment phases and through long-term survivorship is critical. As AYAs age, they will continue to develop and explore sexual identity and sexuality and will become interested in pursuing parenthood and family building. Cancer and treatment-related effects may severely disrupt these processes and alter many aspects that characterize the developmental stages typical of this age range. Sexual and reproductive health issues are essential components of treating the whole person.

The following sections will describe the challenges AYAs face related to their sexual and reproductive health after a cancer diagnosis, provide information for screening patients for heightened distress and dysfunction, and

Table 4.1 Questions to Guide Sexual Health Discussions

Questions to Guide Discussions of Sexual Function and Assess Unmet Needs

Assessment of Current Function

- Are you sexually active or have you been sexually active in the past?
  Note that sexual activities can include . . .
- It is normal for people to experience changes in sexual function and activity as a result of cancer and its treatment. Have you experienced any changes? Have these changes caused problems for you or been distressing?

Assessment of Information Needs

- Do you feel informed about sexual health topics related to cancer treatment effects? Would you like information or recommendations for sexual activity?
- If you are sexually active, are you engaging in safe sex? If so, what do you use?

The use of prophylactics and contraceptives should be assessed to prevent unwanted pregnancy and sexually transmitted infection. For patients on chemotherapy, counseling should be provided about protecting the patient's partner from exposure to chemotherapy.

- Do you have questions about sexual activity after cancer and some of the aids that are available to increase pleasure or reduce any negative symptoms?
- Would you like more information about any of these options?

Provide list of resources or referral to specialists as appropriate.

Assessment of Values and Priorities

- Your psychological health is just as important as your physical health. What is the role of sexuality in your life? Does your current level of sexual activity and sexual pleasure meet your needs?
- How have changes in your sexuality or sex life affected you? What do these changes mean for you?
- Have you experienced any changes in the way you feel about your body, such as body dissatisfaction after cancer? Has this affected you sexually?
- If partnered: How have these changes affected your relationship with your partner? How do you feel about this?
- If single: How have these changes affected your dating or romantic relationships? How do you feel about this?
- Do you think the meaning of sexuality in your culture or religion influences the way you feel about sex?
- How does thinking about these issues make you feel?
- What is most important to you when it comes to your sexuality and experiencing intimacy with another person?

Assessment of Support Needs

- Are you able to experience pleasurable sexual activity and/or experience intimacy with a partner?
- If not, what are some of the barriers and what would be helpful for you?
- Is the support you have received appropriate for your gender identity and sexual orientation?
- Are you interested in sexual aids or sexual intimacy counseling?
- If you have a partner, would they be interested in participating in sexual or intimacy counseling? Is that what you would prefer?
- Do you feel that you have enough support or advice as you continue to explore sexuality after cancer? Do you need more support to navigate these issues?

help clinicians prepare to discuss these complex issues with AYA patients and survivors.

Presenting Problems

Sexual Health

Sexual dysfunction may present in several clinically significant ways, including lack of desire, arousal problems, orgasm problems, pain, and reduced sexual satisfaction (Box 4.1). AYAs with cancers that affect sexual organs may have physical symptoms such as pain even prior to diagnosis, and the continued stress associated with symptoms and diagnosis may further reduce interest in sex even before treatment initiation. During treatment, general side effects impacting energy and physical well-being, such as fatigue, pain, and nausea, are common. Treatments may also affect hormone levels and reduce libido. This is often the case with orchiectomy for testicular cancer in men or hormone therapy that leads to menopausal symptoms in women. In the survivorship phase, AYAs may experience ongoing emotional difficulties that impact sexual function. Negative emotions such as frustration, anger, and sadness, along with unresolved existential feelings resulting from the cancer experience, may lead to lower interest in sexual activity, along with a sense of disconnect from partners and loss of intimacy. These sexual difficulties may impact self-concept in relation to definitions of masculinity and femininity and cause additional distress and avoidance of sexual activity.

Body image is closely related to sexuality and is one of the most pressing difficulties AYAs experience after cancer (Box 4.2). Body image refers to how one feels in relation to the look, feel, and function of one's body. Many aspects of the cancer experience will alter the connection one has to one's body. The diagnosis of cancer itself alters body image, and many survivors describe a sense of betrayal in relation to their body. Physical changes resulting from treatment further affect body image as many patients experience scarring from surgery or radiation, hair loss, placement of a port/central line or stoma, loss of an organ or body part, and weight changes. Understandably,

---

Box 4.1 Sexual Problems

- Pain
- Lack of sexual desire, arousal, interest
- Low libido
- Lower or no sexual activity
- Reduced sexual satisfaction
- **Females**: dyspareunia, vaginal dryness, atrophy, reduced vaginal size, postcoital bleeding, lack of lubrication, premature ovarian insufficiency/menopause
- **Males**: atrophy, erectile dysfunction, orgasmic difficulty, reduced pleasure, painful sex, less energy for sex

> **Box 4.2 Indirect Effects of Cancer Treatment on Sexual Health**
>
> - Negative affect
> - Distress (including depression, anxiety)
> - Negative body image/body mistrust
> - Uncertainty about sequelae of sexual side effects
> - Fatigue and other physical sequelae
> - Relationship worries and concerns; distress about partner's (or potential new partner's) reactions
> - Communication difficulties with partners regarding sexual activity and intimacy
> - Concerns about dating
> - Avoidance of sexual activity (with self or others) and intimacy

experiencing changes in body appearance and functioning will ultimately impact sexuality, including personal connection to body parts and concerns, anxieties, and fears surrounding sexual activity with a partner.

Some patients may cope with cancer-related changes by attempting to disconnect from bodily sensations. Patients have described feeling alienated from their sense of self and body awareness. Feeling disconnected from one's body will undermine sexual feelings and response, which will contribute to or exacerbate sexual problems. Among AYA patients and childhood cancer survivors, the risk of altered body image affecting self-image and sexual intimacy is highest when cancer treatments limit physical growth, cause ongoing physical sequelae, or increase risk of infertility. These issues will often go unresolved if unaddressed and have long-term implications for AYAs' sexuality and sexual well-being in survivorship.

When AYAs experience sexual problems, a sense of social isolation often comes with it. Sexual dysfunction during adolescence and young adulthood is not an experience that survivors easily share with peers. For example, male AYA survivors with erectile dysfunction resulting from treatment may be embarrassed or ashamed, as this is atypical within their age group and likely to be a foreign experience among their peers. For female survivors, symptoms of early menopause or vaginal dryness are also atypical for their younger age and, when combined with the prospect of infertility, may lead to social isolation. It may be difficult for AYAs to seek understanding and support from peers.

Interpersonally, sexual intimacy after cancer presents challenges regarding disclosure and communication with romantic partners or potential new partners. Survivors who are single worry about disclosing their cancer history and sexual problems to a new partner, while those who are partnered may find it difficult to negotiate changes in the relationship both physically and emotionally. Navigating sexual difficulties and conversations with a partner is difficult for many couples, particularly those in new relationships or with limited relationship experience. Given their younger age, AYAs are often single or more informally partnered than older patients facing similar challenges, and their experience in relationships and ability to cope and communicate with partners may be more limited. Within couples, communication difficulties and marital or relationship distress are common consequences of major illness.

Social support from partners may be limited by the extent of patients' (or their partners') psychological maturity, relationship experience, and interest and commitment within the relationship to take on such challenges. AYAs may also be more limited than older adults in their ability to seek help and support, when desired, as they report greater barriers in navigating healthcare systems, accessing treatments, and advocating for needs. Internalized stigma and misperception that these symptoms are not treatable may also prevent AYAs from initiating discussions with healthcare providers.

Reproductive Health

The cancer diagnosis and the type of treatment are the most important factors in contributing to risk of infertility after cancer treatment. Radiation to the gonads and chemotherapy with alkylating agents pose the highest risk; platinum analogues, anthracyclines, and taxanes pose an intermediate risk. Limited evidence is available on newer drugs and therapies, such as immunotherapies, and all patients should be counseled about the possibility of infertility or subfertility after treatment (Box 4.3). Other factors such as age at diagnosis and gonadal functioning prior to diagnosis also play important roles in determining AYA reproductive potential after cancer treatment.

Clinically, it is challenging to quantify the precise risk of infertility associated with individualized treatment regimens, and uncertainty will always be involved in risk estimates. For example, most chemotherapeutic agents are used in combination with other agents, doses vary based on the regimen, and there are increasing numbers of new agents, including targeted and biologic therapies, with minimal long-term data on fertility outcomes. Practically, most treatment protocols will vary from published reports, and it is impossible to predict with certainty how an individual patient will be affected by the treatment and resulting reproductive potential.

Male AYA patients receiving cancer treatment may develop impaired semen production from depletion of the spermatogonial stem cell population or impaired sperm transport secondary to erectile or ejaculatory dysfunction. Female AYA patients may experience premature ovarian failure from depletion of follicles or may not be able to carry a pregnancy secondary to radiation-induced uterine fibrosis or hysterectomy. Although some women may have preserved ovarian function, diminished ovarian reserve may still occur, putting them at risk for premature menopause (i.e., premature ovarian

---

Box 4.3 Fertility Problems

- Irregular menstrual cycles
- Hormonal imbalances and menopausal symptoms
- Active hormone replacement therapy
- Established diagnosis of primary hypogonadism

failure), health effects of altered hormone levels, or risks with carrying a pregnancy.

Surgical procedures that affect reproductive organs will also impact fertility and reproductive potential. For males, surgical treatment for testicular, colon, bladder, or prostate cancer may impair sperm production and/or cause ejaculatory dysfunction. For women, treatment for gynecologic cancers may include removal of one or both ovaries and partial or complete removal of fallopian tubes, uterus, vagina, or cervix.

Radiation targeting the abdominal area, including reproductive organs, the bladder, large intestines, and rectum, may affect a man's sperm production or impair a woman's ability to safely carry a pregnancy to term or affect the ovaries and follicle count.

Cranial surgery or irradiation that involves the pituitary gland may lead to disruption of the hypothalamic–pituitary–gonadal axis that regulates sperm production and oocyte maturation.

Clinicians should note if female patients report irregular menstrual cycles. Reports of reduced libido may also be indicative of hormonal imbalances and have implications for reproductive health.

However, the presence or absence of menstruation is not an absolute indicator of fecundity.

Young women may experience transient chemotherapy-induced amenorrhea lasting up to 3 years after treatment, though most resume menses within 24 months. Likewise, hormone levels used to evaluate fertility, such as antimüllerian hormone (AMH), have been shown to fluctuate as a side effect of cancer treatment, with some evidence showing possible recovery of AMH levels in the few years after treatment. Patients may incorrectly interpret a lack of menstruation or abnormal hormone levels as an indicator of infertility and worry unnecessarily or, conversely, they may assume normative ovarian reserve and reproductive potential with the presence of menstruation. For AYAs who are interested in future family building involving personal gametes to have a biologically related child, a fertility evaluation by a fertility specialist (reproductive endocrinologist) is recommended for comprehensive testing and appropriate counseling.

Besides the physical determination of reproductive health, (risk of) infertility often leads to a number of psychosocial and emotional difficulties for AYA survivors, including distress about achieving parenthood, worries about dating and romantic partners' expectations or reactions, and comparison to peers (Box 4.4). Fertility-related concerns may include difficulty coping with uncertainty about reproductive potential and timeline, particularly among single women and women struggling with perceived time pressures associated with "biological clocks."

It is common for AYAs to worry about passing on a genetic risk for cancer to a future child. For some survivors, the experience of cancer causes a sense of "body mistrust," and women in particular question whether their bodies are strong enough to handle a pregnancy or fear recurrence during pregnancy.

> **Box 4.4 How Fertility Concerns May Present**
>
> - Distress (including depression, anxiety)
> - Uncertainty about reproductive potential and family-building options
> - Fear of being unable to achieve parenthood
> - For women, anxiety about "biological clocks" and reproductive time window
> - Concerns about passing on a genetic risk for cancer to a future child
> - Negative body image/body mistrust; fears about pregnancy
> - Relationship worries and concerns; distress about partner's (or potential new partner's) reactions and fear of rejection
> - Concerns about dating and disclosure
> - Avoidance of fertility information or evaluation as a way to cope with distress (e.g., fear of receiving bad news)
> - Feeling "left behind" as peers begin to have children; distress about delayed family building and unmet expectations for life goals

Related psychosocial concerns include worries about dating and disclosure, communicating with partners, and difficulty with the social aspects of pursuing family building as friends begin to have children and celebrate parenthood. Attending others' baby showers may be difficult for AYAs to cope with.

Survivors may face great uncertainty stemming from the exact nature of infertility risk, lack of knowledge about how to obtain fertility care, uncertainty about options for having children, and questions about personal priorities, values, and goals related to family-building options. Uncertainty about the process and outcomes of pursuing parenthood may be highly anxiety-provoking and challenging to cope with. Many AYAs are uninformed about alternative family-building options and will likely have questions about processes involved and factors to consider in making decisions about family building via IVF, surrogacy, use of donor gametes, and/or adoption (international or domestic).

Assessment

Whenever possible, the assessment of sexual health and fertility outcomes should include review of medical charts and consulting with the treating oncology team. It can be helpful to incorporate information from specialists with insight on treatment-specific effects, including oncologists, gynecologists or urologists, and reproductive endocrinologists.

Additional steps in the assessment process may include use of validated instruments to more formally measure patient-reported outcomes. Measures designed to assess sexual dysfunction and reproductive concerns are helpful, particularly combined with a more global assessment of well-being such as depressive and anxiety symptoms or quality-of-life domains. Quality-of-life measures developed for AYAs affected by cancer include a range of domains including physical, cognitive, emotional, social, and spiritual functioning. There have been four quality-of-life measures developed that cover sexual health and/or intimate relationships, and three include fertility concerns.[5] These may be used to quantify the psychosocial concerns of AYAs and facilitate clinical assessment, inform ensuing conversations, and/or track change over time or progress in therapy. Selection of measures may be guided by the target age of patients within the AYA age range, as some tools were validated with adolescents, whereas others were validated in an older AYA age group. Assessment tools may also be useful for understanding how concerns about sexual and reproductive health fit within the broader context of adjusting to cancer and survivorship.

Scripts for clinicians have also been published to guide discussions with AYAs pertaining to sexual problems and fertility concerns.[6,7]

Sexual Health

Assessing the onset, duration, and impact of sexual dysfunction should be done using standardized instruments in addition to semistructured clinical interview. Aubin and Perez provide a "clinician's toolbox" to assess the sexual impact of cancer specifically designed for the assessment and treatment of AYA patients.[8] Their approach offers a useful structure for clinical assessment, which can be complemented by questionnaires and treatment approaches that are tailored based on gender and disease group.

While many scales have been developed, the choice of a self-report inventory of sexual symptoms should be based on its relevance to a particular patient. The most clinically meaningful assessment tools will investigate both physical symptoms and their emotional impact. It is important for the clinician to clarify with patients whether or not they are interested in resuming sexual activity (if stopped) and identify patient-driven goals for recovery during the assessment process.

For women, one of the most commonly used self-administered measures is the Female Sexual Function Index (FSFI), which includes subscales assessing problems with desire, arousal, lubrication, orgasm, satisfaction, and pain. The FSFI has been validated in patients with cancer and cancer survivors, and a breast cancer–specific adaptation of the FSFI (FSFI-BC) also exists. Similarly, the Arizona Sexual Experiences Scale (ASEX) includes multidimensional assessment of sexual problems with similar subscales as the FSFI, though it is less widely used. The FSFI and ASEX were identified in a systematic review as tools that have acceptable psychometric properties in patients with breast cancer. Other measures include the Sexual Function Questionnaire (SFQ), the Brief Sexual Symptom Checklist for Women, and the Gynecologic Leiden Questionnaire. To assess distress related to sexual dysfunction specifically, there is the Female Sexual Distress—Revised scale. To screen and diagnose hypoactive sexual desire disorder, the Decreased Sexual Desire Screening may be used.

For men, the International Index of Erectile Function (IIEF) is a commonly used measure and is available in 15 languages. Other self-administered measures include the Sexual Health Inventory for Men and the Sexual Quality of Life Questionnaire—Men. The Male Sexual Health Questionnaire—Ejaculatory Dysfunction Scale is a screening and outcome measure for ejaculatory dysfunction and bother related to ejaculation specifically.

For both males and females, the PROMIS Sexual Function and Satisfaction Measures Brief Profile is a good option that includes male- and female-specific questions. The measure provides scores on seven subdomains of sexual function: interest in sexual activity, vaginal discomfort (women only), lubrication (women only), erectile function (men only), orgasm, and global satisfaction with sex life. One of the advantages of the PROMIS measures is the free scoring system and translation of scores to compare to population-level data.

While scales tailored to non–gender-conforming populations are not currently available, generalized scales such as the Short Sexual Functioning Scale or the ASEX offer overviews of function that apply generally. If a particular gendered scale is preferred based on its content, a clinician should allow patients to elect which form, if any, they feel most comfortable completing. Notably, to inform care, clinicians should be aware of patients' anatomic body parts, as these may differ from self-identified gender. For example, vaginal health concerns may still be an issue for a patient who presents as male but who has a vagina, and care should be taken to connect patients with appropriate care and recommendations.

Body image scales can be used across genders to assess for the impact of body and self-image on sexual functioning. A generalized body image scale, developed to measure body image concerns after cancer, has also been modified to enable use and comparison to healthy controls. It incorporates items about physical attractiveness and body perceptions.

When interpreting standardized assessments of sexual functioning, clinicians should consider contextual factors that may inadvertently skew scores. For example, scores indicating low levels of sexual activity may reflect sexual dysfunction or unrelated factors such as the unavailability of a partner. It is important to clarify reasons for sexual inactivity in particular and identify goals of recovery. Based on their health literacy and emotional reactions to these assessments, some AYAs may leave questions blank, indicating discomfort or confusion rather than sexual dysfunction. Clinicians should consider reviewing standardized assessments with patients; this can also provide a forum for providing information and discussing any sexual health concerns.

Reproductive Health

All patients of reproductive age should be asked about their interest in future family building and desire to receive counseling about infertility risks associated with treatment. Assessment of parenthood interest and desire to learn about fertility-preservation options may follow.

After treatment, referral for a fertility evaluation by a reproductive endocrinologist should be made for all AYAs who are worried about or interested in learning about their fertility status. Whenever possible, referral to fertility specialists with experience treating cancer survivors and knowledge of transient treatment effects and optimal timing for evaluation is ideal. For survivors who are not yet ready to have a child and may not need comprehensive counseling about family-building options, a urologist, gynecologist, or primary care physician may be able to test hormone levels and provide some information on current fertility status.

Assessment of fertility will include testing of hormone levels and, for women, a pelvic ultrasound to assess the structure of reproductive organs. A reproductive endocrinologist should complete this assessment and may provide counseling on family-building options after treatment, including the likelihood of success using reproductive medicine to achieve pregnancy, such as with IVF with fresh, frozen, or donated gametes. Some patients should not pursue pregnancy if there are safety concerns about elevated hormone levels, carrying a fetus to full term, or risks for cancer recurrence during pregnancy, and oncology providers should provide recommendations.

The assessment of fertility problems should include a medical evaluation of fertility and reproductive potential, as well as an evaluation of the patient's knowledge of fertility and reproductive health topics and psychosocial difficulties. AYAs will have varying levels of knowledge about reproductive health and personal fertility status and reproductive potential.

Clinicians should remember that not all AYAs will desire parenthood or be interested in future childbearing.

Questions to assess patients' level of interest in receiving fertility information and counseling may be used to initiate discussions, such as, "*Do you hope to have children in the future?*" (Table 4.2). Following this, further evaluation of the type and nature of concerns, if any, may be warranted.

The Oncofertility Consortium of Northwestern University (www.oncofertility.northwestern.edu) provides a number of assessment tools for providers to use in the context of cancer and fertility care, including male and female onco-fertility decision trees, assessment and discussion algorithms and discussion guidelines, and an adolescent values-clarification tool.

For female survivors, the Reproductive Concerns After Cancer Scale (RCACS) is an 18-item scale made up of six subdomains of fertility-related difficulties, including concerns about fertility potential, partner disclosure, the health of a future child, personal health, and achieving pregnancy, as well as the degree of acceptance of cancer-related fertility problems. The authors of the RCACS, Gorman et al., have also presented preliminary data on the development of a parallel male version of the scale, including items that cover the same six subdomains, but at the time of writing this scale has not been published. Another scale for female survivors is the Reproductive Concerns Scale, which measures various aspects of fertility-related concern but is not cancer-specific.

For adolescent patients, careful attention should be paid to the use of parental reports as proxy measures for adolescent concerns. Quinn et al. conducted research using the Reproductive Concerns Instrument to assess fertility-related concerns of female adolescents (aged 12 to 18 years old)

Table 4.2 Questions to Guide Fertility Discussions

Questions to Guide Fertility Discussions and Assess Decision Support Needs

Assessment of Interest
- Have you considered whether you would like to have children in the future?
- What are your hopes and goals for family building?
- (If children are wanted) What is your anticipated timeline/how far or near in the future would you want to have children?

Assessment of Information Needs
- What is your understanding about how your cancer treatment may affect (has affected) your ability to have children?
- Would you like to know more about how your fertility can be evaluated?
- Have you considered other options to have a child (e.g., using donor sperm, gestational carrier [with embryo created from patient's egg or donor eggs] or adoption)?
- Would you like more information about any of these options?

Provide list of resources as appropriate

Assessment of Values and Priorities
- Your personal feelings are just as important as medical facts. Have you thought about how important it is to you to have a biologic child or to experience pregnancy as opposed to using donor eggs/sperm, using a gestational carrier, or adoption?
- What would it mean for you if you were unable to attempt pregnancy?
- What are your major concerns, and how does thinking about these issues make you feel?

Assessment of Support Needs
- Do you feel confident that you can make a decision about how you want to pursue family building when you are ready to? If not, what would be helpful for you as you consider this decision?
- Is there someone else you are making this decision with? To what extent are you in agreement about your options to have a child?
- Do you feel that you have other people in your life you can turn to for support or advice as you think about this decision?

and their parents. The results of this research suggested that quality-of-life instruments may not be adequate for capturing younger patients' concerns and parent-proxy reports were not accurate. Findings provide further evidence about the importance of clinical conversations when assessing fertility concerns and reproductive health issues, particularly for younger AYAs.

For AYAs with confirmed infertility and those experiencing infertility-related problems, the FertiQoL was developed by an international collaboration that included the American Society for Reproductive Medicine and the European Society of Human Reproduction and Embryology. It is a validated measure to assess the quality of life of individuals experiencing fertility problems and may be used independent of infertility treatment status. The scale measures the physical, emotional, and relational challenges associated with fertility problems, with additional questions to evaluate the impact of infertility treatment on quality of life for those undergoing infertility treatment (e.g., treatment tolerability).

Considerations for Differential Diagnosis

While it is difficult to reliably predict the extent of treatment-related effects on sexual and reproductive health, it is expected that different types of cancer treatment will lead to different symptoms and outcomes. For young males, cancer treatments that affect the testicles or the pituitary gland may affect the production and circulation of testosterone, which may hinder sexual development and can be treated by prescribed exogenous testosterone. For young females, radiation or chemotherapy to the ovaries or radiation to the pituitary gland may affect sexual development and fertility, and necessitate hormone replacement therapy.

Given the different biology of the male and female reproductive system, defining reproductive health among male and female AYA survivors is rather complex. Female survivors may experience premature ovarian insufficiency, which indicates that the ovarian reserve is depleted and survivors are infertile; or survivors may show signs of reduced ovarian reserve, which typically indicates that they are still fertile at present, but may experience menopause earlier than would be expected for normative populations without cancer. Importantly, for those with a lowered ovarian reserve, natural conception may still be possible, but the window of reproductive viability may be shorter. These patients may be counseled to consider fertility preservation after treatment to mitigate risks of premature ovarian failure (early menopause) if they were unable to preserve fertility prior to treatment. Other survivors may be relatively unaffected by treatments and have a preserved reproductive timeline similar to age-matched populations.

Male survivors' reproductive health can be characterized through semen analysis, which may show azoospermia, indicating that no sperm is present in the ejaculate (sterility); oligo-/asthenospermia, if the sperm count is severely reduced or the form or activity of semen is abnormal; or normospermia, indicating that the reproductive system is unharmed.

For both sexual and reproductive health, an important differential diagnosis when treating AYA patients and survivors will be to identify clinically significant levels of distress and appropriately characterize sources of distress. Evidence suggests that both sexual dysfunction and infertility increase the risk for depression and anxiety, particularly if sexual symptoms are unresolved in survivorship and/or if survivors are unable to achieve parenthood.

Clinical Management

Sexual Health

AYAs often wish to talk about sexual problems and strategies to improve sexual health with their healthcare providers yet are reluctant to bring these topics up.

Clinicians should be prepared to initiate such discussions and ensure confidentiality for AYAs, following legal regulations for what age constitutes minors and minors' rights in healthcare settings.

Clinicians should bring up sexual health as a standard part of cancer care, particularly in the context of providing psychosocial support for the myriad of quality-of-life difficulties that result from cancer and treatment. The tone of such discussions should be open, nonjudgmental, collaborative, and direct. For some AYAs, it may be necessary to be cautious introducing the topic of sexuality and sexual dysfunction, depending on clinical judgment about patients' interest and readiness to have such discussions and sensitivity to their level of sexual development and experience. Clinicians should be prepared to discuss sexual health topics with AYAs who identify as gender nonconforming or as gender/sexual minorities, including lesbian, gay, bisexual, transgender, questioning, or intersex (LGBTQI) (see Chapter 3).

Normalize Discussing Sexuality

When raising these issues, the clinician should start from a foundation of trust and rapport with the patient. One of the first goals in providing treatment should be to normalize the experience of sexual dysfunction. Equally important, clinicians should validate patients' experiences and concerns and provide empathy. It is important to be knowledgeable about national and local resources and age-appropriate referrals to offer patients based on their needs and long-term goals. In some cases, a patient may wish to discuss sexual concerns with a nurse, mental health counselor, or interventionist rather than with a doctor; such preferences should be accommodated by training and equipping all practitioners with skills to discuss these matters and having clinician resources readily available to aid conversations and appropriate referral.

Offer Anticipatory Guidance

At present, it is estimated that a minority of AYA patients are offered guidance on cancer-related sexual health issues before treatment, yet all patients would likely benefit from preparatory discussions and opportunity to ask questions. Anticipatory management to prepare patients for sexual side effects should include education to set expectations and prepare for body changes, along with an introduction to coping and treatment measures if difficulties arise. Topics covered in these early conversations should then be integrated into the early stages of cancer treatment as side effects and bodily changes begin to occur and challenges are more fully realized by patients.

Offer Ongoing "Check-ins"

Ongoing "check-in" discussions throughout active treatment stages will ensure patients have an opportunity to ask questions and receive help when needed. The goal is to provide care at the point of need to avoid more serious problems from developing and to mitigate broader effects on psychosocial well-being. Patients may still be interested in sexual activity and intimacy but have questions about safety and treatment-related risks. Providing the opportunity to have discussions and a safe place to ask questions is vitally important so that patients can "opt in" to having discussions and accessing care if and when they are ready.

Broaden Definitions of Sex and Intimacy

Clinical discussions should stress that sexual intimacy is much more than penetrative intercourse and a range of activities may help to maintain intimacy and emotional closeness among partners, even during active treatment or when physical well-being is low. Sexual problem solving may help AYAs to discover new ways of achieving physical intimacy, pleasure, and emotional closeness with a partner, despite experiencing body changes with treatment. Finding new sexual positions that are comfortable and/or nonpenetrative activities that are pleasurable and satisfying will help couples maintain closeness. For example, positions that allow women to control the depth or angle of penetration may be helpful. Counseling should encourage patients to be open to new sexual activities and prompt couples to be creative and work together to think of new ways to be intimate.

Treatment for sexual problems should take a biopsychosocial approach to address the multidimensional nature of sexuality and intimacy. Discussions and resources provided to AYA survivors should be appropriate and tailored based on age, sexual orientation, and cultural or religious beliefs. Information about sexual health should be delivered more than once, with sensitivity to the developmental readiness of an AYA patient to receive and act on the resources provided.

Include Gynecologic Care

AYA survivors who are avoiding sexual activity after cancer may also avoid gynecologic care if they fear that pelvic exams will cause pain. Avoidance of gynecologic care has important health implications for female patients, regardless of sexual function. Particularly for survivors at elevated risk of recurrence or secondary gynecologic cancer, addressing vaginal health symptoms and supporting vaginal recovery (such as with dilator therapy), while providing education on the importance of adhering to medical care recommendations and psychological support, may be warranted.

Provide Psychoeducation

Psychoeducation about how treatment-related effects may impact sexual function is a necessary first step. Patients' concerns and experiences should be normalized, and empathic listening and support should be provided.

- A description of sexual anatomy and functioning may be needed. AYAs may be uninformed about the sexual response cycle, so education can help them understand their difficulties and appropriate treatment strategies.

- Providers may provide informational resources to guide discussions, introduce the use of sexual aids, and/or make referrals to sex therapists as needed. Many problems may be solved with a problem-solving approach such as exploring new sexual positions to avoid pain.

- Communication skills training may help patients navigate discussions with their partners, particularly if sexual topics are viewed as embarrassing or shameful.

- Addressing maladaptive cognitions and reframing negative beliefs that undermine recovery should be a part of therapy as needed.

- In most instances, it is important to include partners in therapy, if desired by the patient. Partners can offer insight about their experiences, concerns, and needs. Incorporating partners in treatment may also help to alleviate the burden on patients to navigate conversations with their partners or relay instructions and recommendations.

- Consulting a sex therapist can offer a forum for patients or couples to discuss their concerns, desires, and goals related to their sexuality and sexual relationships, particularly if first-line treatments are not adequate and if more significant sexual problems are experienced.

The duration and phase of treatment may shape sexual behavior and clinical recommendations. Patients may need to suspend some sexual activities and/or penetrative intercourse during the treatment phase for some disease groups and treatments. Vaginal and anal penetration are discouraged after surgery to the pelvic area and after chemotherapy treatments that lower white blood cell count, leading to immunosuppression, low platelet count, and associated risk of bleeding. Patients may still desire physical intimacy, however, and modifying behaviors to maintain intimacy should be discussed. Active treatment often causes side effects such as nausea, low energy, and fatigue, which will impact sexual function. Patients may still desire physical intimacy and closeness with a partner. Other patients may cope with treatment side effects on their own and withdraw from sexual activity and intimacy. During maintenance therapy and the survivorship phase, resuming sexual activity may be complicated by ongoing side effects, concerns about body image, and unresolved psychological and emotional issues related to the cancer experience. Negative feelings may persist or worsen in the transition to survivorship and continue for years. For those who were diagnosed with cancer in childhood and are now AYAs, late effects of treatment can affect sexual development and sexual function with ongoing physical and emotional challenges as a survivor.

Interventions to improve sexual function in AYA cancer survivors should begin with the least complex and least invasive approaches. Any therapy, including pharmacologic, mechanical, or psychotherapeutic approaches, should be tailored to the sexual preference of the AYA survivor. In many cases, therapeutic approaches will be similar irrespective of gender and sexual identity; treating erectile dysfunction or body image concerns for men who have sex with men will be similar to that of heterosexual partners and likewise for women who have sex with women. Notably, the clinician should be aware of gender identity in relation to biologic sex: not all patients who present as women may have a vagina and not all patients who present as men will have a penis. Counseling should take place in a nonjudgmental and sex-positive frame. Even when oncology care providers are not prepared to comprehensively address sexual dysfunction treatments, they should routinely screen for sexual health symptoms, concerns, and questions among AYA survivors to provide appropriate referrals for specialized care.

Sexual Health Clinical Management for Female AYAs

First-line treatments include nonhormonal approaches for managing urogenital symptoms or atrophy-related urinary symptoms.

Nonhormonal vaginal moisturizers may be used to reduce vaginal dryness and should be applied every few days or multiple times per week.

Lubricants may be used during intercourse to help with dryness, irritation, and pain.

These localized treatments have targeted efficacy with minimal side effects. Water- and silicone-based products, available over the counter, are preferable to petroleum-based products, which may interfere with the effectiveness of condoms. Topical vitamin E oil can also relieve dryness. If moisturizers and lubricants do not address the problem, and for patients unresponsive to non-hormonal remedies, low-dose vaginal estrogen therapy to treat urogenital symptoms and vulvovaginal atrophy is highly effective. It is administered as a vaginal ring or tablet by prescription. For patients with hormone-dependent breast cancer, using tablets or the ring to administer treatment is better than creams.

Vaginal dilators may be used if women experience vaginal atrophy. They mechanically stretch the vagina to improve elasticity and reduce dyspareunia.

Although dilators have shown to be effective, adherence is low and many patients never initiate use or discontinue use. Treatment is stepwise and may lead to frustration in the intermittent stages, necessitating adequate education about proper use and support from clinicians.

Kegel exercises, during which women tense and relax their pelvic floor muscles at regular intervals, may be beneficial, as regularly exercising the pelvic floor muscles can improve control and thereby facilitate relaxation of muscles surrounding the vaginal entrance, urethra, and anus to reduce tension and subsequent pain during sexual activity and intercourse. They can be done daily.

Kegel exercises can be augmented by specialized physical therapy, which can provide pelvic biofeedback to help optimize localization to the muscles that will facilitate sexual recovery and allow women to reduce muscle tension during sexual activity, which is often the source of pain or exacerbates discomfort. Referral to a pelvic health specialist may be warranted.

Hormonal approaches to sexual dysfunction among women include low-dose estrogen therapy to address vaginal atrophy or testosterone therapy to address reduced libido.[9] The use of hormonal therapy for sexual dysfunction remains controversial due in part to hormone-sensitive cancers and the risk of development of secondary neoplasms, and many patients may refuse treatments because they have heard of risks whether evidence-based or not. Newer research suggests localized hormone therapies do not increase risks. However, patients may still be concerned and education about this research may be necessary to alleviate their fears. An informed decision-making and consent process should be taken in which patients are educated about potential risks and benefits of low-dose vaginal estrogen so they can make an informed choice. Oncology providers may need to be consulted. Treatment plans should be guided by evidence-based strategies aligned with patient preferences.

Sexual Health Clinical Management for Male AYAs

First-line treatment for male sexual problems often focuses on addressing erectile dysfunction and the emotional difficulties that arise with a perceived loss of masculinity.

Phosphodiesterase type 5 (PDE5) inhibitors are oral medications and represent the general first-line approach for the treatment of erectile dysfunction. PDE5 inhibitors act to amplify the normal erectile physiology. Their success depends on intact libido, sexual stimulation, sensory pathways, and other factors that are required for erectile function.

They are not effective for all patients, and efficacy is further reduced by poor adherence to intake instructions (i.e., take on an empty stomach, 2 hours before sexual intercourse). Many men discontinue their use despite continued distress about erectile difficulties and lack of sexual recovery.

Vacuum erectile devices (VEDs) or penile injections may also be used. VEDs represent a mechanical means of causing erection by pulling blood into the penis. It is recommended that erection by this method, which includes a rubber ring to sustain it, be kept for a maximum of 30 minutes. The erection may differ in appearance and function from a spontaneous erection. Daily use of the VED is recommended to prevent penis length loss, and practitioners training AYA survivors in the use of the VED may emphasize its function in improving sexual response and preventing genital changes.

Intracavernosal injection at the base of the penis can be used to improve sexual response by dilating blood vessels to pull in blood flow. It takes effect in approximately 10 minutes and the ensuring erection lasts up to 30 minutes. Men who are prescribed this therapy are coached by a urologist or other specialist in self-administering injections, which are described as minimally painful. Despite its effectiveness, many men do not like the idea of doing injections. Counseling should be provided to support men in adjusting to the idea of this treatment, as it may be highly effective. For men unable to self-administer intracavernosal injections, intraurethral suppositories with similar mechanisms of action may be used but are generally less effective.

For men who do not respond to medical, mechanical, or injection therapy, surgery to install an inflatable penile prosthesis is available and highly effective.

Sexuality and Intimacy

Given the interplay of physical and psychological factors in sexual intimacy, sexual dysfunction may best be addressed in a holistic manner. Intercourse may not be possible for some survivors after cancer, and alternative activities that are still sexually satisfying should be part of sexual rehabilitation. For survivors who are partnered, intimacy can be maintained without intercourse through practices such as nonsexual touching. Sensation-focused exercises and positive body awareness and touching may be pleasurable activities for individuals or couples without the added pressure (and fear) of sexual activity leading to intercourse with penetration. This may be the case if the survivor is worried about experiencing pain or discomfort or does not feel emotionally ready for intercourse. For example, sensuous massage and "outer-course" (such as kissing or touching body parts) can alleviate the pressure to perform sexually while still feeling stimulation and maintaining intimacy with a partner. Sex practices that include oral or clitoral stimulation may provide approaches to sexual pleasure without penetration or if erectile dysfunction or vaginal pain is an issue.

Body image concerns about hair loss, weight changes, and scarring may be especially distressing for AYAs because of their association with premature aging and deviation from societal norms of body ideals, including beliefs about a "thin ideal" for women and "muscular ideal" for men. Counseling should be sensitive to these concerns and normalize body changes in the context of cancer treatment.

For AYAs who are single and those concerned about how their partner might react to changes in their sexual performance and/or physical appearance, self-stimulation can provide sexual gratification and help identify what is pleasurable. Providers can address and try to reduce stigma related to masturbation and endorse the use of certain devices and sexual aids. Discussing and facilitating self-gratification may also be appropriate for younger survivors, who may be sexually inexperienced and wish to build knowledge and comfort with their own sexual feelings and sensations.

Psychosocial Support

Providing psychosocial support to promote sexual health in AYA survivors entails normalizing sexual symptoms and emphasizing their treatability, validating concerns about sexual health and its impact on relationships, and formulating strategies targeted to particular sexual symptoms or priorities in a relationship.

Cognitive-Behavioral Therapy

Cognitive-behavioral approaches may be used to address emotional difficulties and maladaptive beliefs contributing to sexual problems and guide the development of more positive coping strategies. For example, cognitions surrounding fear of failure and performance anxiety in men with erectile dysfunction often undermine the success of treatment and must be addressed before treatments may be used with success. Cognitions related to negative body image, such as among women who have undergone mastectomies or patients who have altered body functioning, will also exacerbate sexual difficulties and undermine treatments and recovery. Cognitive-behavioral therapy may include the AYA survivor alone or with a partner, depending on the clinical presentation and the identified factors that are maintaining sexual problems. Clinicians may choose to have individual sessions with each member of a couple, followed by joint sessions to review the couple's experiences, establish goals of therapy, and initiate treatment. Although cancer treatment effects may have caused sexual problems, psychosocial and emotional factors may be key factors preventing recovery. It is important that treatments incorporate these factors to optimize recovery.

Safer Sex Practices

Treating AYAs should include an open dialogue and discussion about safer sex practices and advising patients not to take sexual risks. Acquiring sexually transmitted diseases is particularly risky for AYA survivors who have a compromised immune system, and they should be made aware of this increased risk. Of note, there may be poor sexual health literacy in this age group, particularly if AYAs missed school-based health education due to illness-related disruptions. Basic education about sexual and reproductive anatomy and safer sexual practices may be warranted.

Use of prophylactics during intercourse is vital to protect survivors against sexually transmitted infection. For example, acquiring human papillomavirus (HPV) could increase the survivor's risk for HPV-related cancers in addition to an elevated susceptibility to second malignancies following an initial cancer diagnosis. Patients who remain sexually active during the treatment phase should use a condom to prevent exposing a partner to chemotherapy through vaginal or oral excretion.

Contraception

Lower adherence to contraception has been reported among AYA survivors of childhood cancer and may be linked to a lack of awareness of fertility status. Female survivors were found to use emergency contraception at higher rates than their same-age peers. Based on the type of chemotherapy treatment, pregnancy is discouraged and may be unsafe for a specified period of time—often for at least 2 years, though patients should seek guidance from their oncologist. Within a treatment team, it may be optimal for multiple clinicians to provide information and counseling to ensure that patients are adequately informed and adhering to recommendations about contraception.

Reproductive Health

Initiating developmentally appropriate conversations and providing the opportunity for patients (and/or partners or parents) to ask questions and access specialized fertility care is a critical aspect of treating AYA patients. Clinicians should refer to guidelines put forward by professional organizations to guide clinical management, including oncology and reproductive medicine societies such as the American Society of Clinical Oncology (ASCO), the European Society for Medical Oncology (ESMO), the Clinical Oncology Society of Australia (COSA), the American Society of Reproductive Medicine (ASRM), and the European Society of Human Reproduction and Embryology (ESHRE).

Advances in reproductive technology have given patients options for preserving fertility potential. These include techniques to freeze gametes (sperm, eggs, or embryos) or gonadal tissue (cryopreservation) and strategies to reduce the gonadal toxicity of cancer treatments.

Not all AYA patients will be interested in future family building or fertility preservation. Others may be interested, but the need to initiate cancer treatment may preclude options. This is particularly true for women because oocyte/embryo cryopreservation takes at least 10 to 14 days. For those who are interested, fertility preservation should ideally be completed before treatment initiation as even a single treatment with gonadotoxic therapy can affect gamete quality and DNA integrity.

For postpubertal males, sperm banking is standard of care for fertility preservation, and most patients obtain semen by masturbation. For males who are unable to collect semen by masturbation, electro-ejaculation or testicular sperm extraction may be alternative options, while testicular shielding may also be done for those undergoing radiation with potential testicular exposure.

For postpubertal females, standard options are egg freezing and embryo freezing with a partner's or donated sperm.

For females unable or unwilling to delay treatment for 2 weeks to complete cryopreservation, ovarian tissue cryopreservation (with future transplantation) may be an option. Although still considered experimental, at the time of this writing, over 130 live births have been reported worldwide, with a 26% live-birth success rate, with some indication that there may even be scenarios in which freezing ovarian tissue is preferable to freezing eggs.[10] Other options to minimize gonadal damage include ovarian transposition, ovarian suppression, pelvic shielding, and modifications in the cancer treatment plan, all of which are also considered experimental at this time.

Prepubertal patients have limited options for fertility preservation, and all are considered experimental. This may leave many survivors of childhood cancer infertile, and it is important to consider their concerns as they are often overlooked by parents and providers. Studies have shown that prepubertal patients have desires and intentions about achieving parenthood and are concerned about treatment-related fertility impairment. As with sexual health counseling, clinicians should obtain permission from parents to have private conversations with underage patients to discuss treatment effects and fertility-preservation options in a developmentally appropriate manner and based on the patient's readiness to have such discussions. Discussions and educational resources need to be tailored to the patient's age, maturity, and perceived readiness to have such discussions.

All patients of reproductive age should be informed about infertility risks associated with treatments and have the opportunity to consider fertility preservation before treatment begins.

At the time of diagnosis, patients may be overwhelmed by the sudden life disruption brought on by a cancer diagnosis and whirlwind of treatment planning. Nevertheless, most patients say they desire fertility-related information at this time and want to be informed of risks. Patients who are provided fertility counselling are less likely to experience future distress and regret compared to those who do not receive counseling, even when fertility preservation is not pursued. Conversely, AYAs have reported feeling "dismissed" by oncology teams regarding their fertility-related concerns, and those who feel ignored or invalidated may refrain from asking further questions yet continue to worry. If fertility preservation is possible, patients may need support in making decisions about whether to pursue such options or how to overcome barriers such as seeking financial assistance or applying for patient grants to help with high costs.

🔍 Referral to a fertility specialist (reproductive endocrinologist) is typically an important first step for patients to access specialized testing and counseling both before and after treatment.

🔍 Conversations should be developmentally appropriate depending on the patient's age, maturity, and readiness to think about topics surrounding fertility and family building. Older survivors may be better equipped to cope with infertility risks and distress and more motivated to obtain information. On the other hand, even younger AYAs report fears and worry about future reproductive potential, and clinicians should be prepared to have such discussions even in pediatric settings.

🔍 Addressing concerns about fertility and family-building intentions in the context of cancer care should be an ongoing process throughout the cancer care trajectory.

Survivors have consistently reported a preference for clinicians to proactively address fertility before, during, and after treatment. AYAs should be provided opportunities to ask questions, complete fertility assessments, and receive support and early referral if and when desired. Checking in with AYAs periodically during treatment and as a routine part of survivorship care is important to assess whether their interest or concerns have changed. As AYAs age, the nature of their concerns will evolve, and priorities will change. Clinicians providing ongoing support will need to respond to their changing needs for information. Clinicians should not make judgments about AYAs' interest in learning about fertility and family building based on age, and periodic check-ins will help to identify appropriate times to have such discussions. In posttreatment survivorship, having early and ongoing discussions may also facilitate mourning and acceptance around the loss of fertility, while allowing time to adjust to alternative family-building options and build hope that parenthood is still possible.

Resources
Informational materials are often helpful to aid clinical discussions. Adolescents tend to prefer online educational materials and support, whereas parents have reported a preference for informational booklets. Often, offering information in the form of pamphlets or booklets, combined with referrals to trusted information that can be accessed online at patients' (or parents') convenience, is best. Information should be offered during in-person conversations to introduce the topic, answer any questions, and provide counseling and referral as needed. Patients who are interested and able to pursue fertility preservation should be referred to a reproductive endocrinologist.

Many resources for clinicians to use and/or provide to their patients are available online, including educational pamphlets, provider pocket guides (including links to smartphone apps freely available for download), and fertility decision tree tools from trusted organizations such as the Oncofertility Consortium of Northwestern University, LIVESTRONG Fertility, and SaveMyFertility.org. Providers may also access online databases to find a local fertility specialist through the American Society for Reproductive Medicine (www.reproductivefacts.org) and Alliance for Fertility Preservation (www.allianceforfertilitypreservation.org). The Oncofertility Consortium has published a fertility values clarification tool for adolescent females diagnosed with cancer that includes instructions and guidelines for providers (available free for download), along with other resources for both patients and providers.

Decision Support

At the time of this writing, nine decision aids have been developed by clinical researchers to support AYAs in making decisions about fertility preservation prior to treatment; most are aimed at female patients considering egg/embryo freezing. The purpose of decision aids is to help patients understand their options; communicate their concerns, needs, and priorities; and ultimately make "values-based decisions" that are in line with their priorities and goals. Decision aids typically provide information about the decision options, offer guidance around risk/benefit tradeoffs, and include values-clarification exercises to help patients identify personal values and relate values to decision options. Some decision aids guide patients in engaging providers, encouraging shared decision-making. The Ottawa Hospital Research Institute is a rich source of information and resources for providers to use to guide patients in making values-based decisions, including evidence-based guidelines, decision aid templates and examples, evaluation measures, and decision coaching tools (www.decisionaid.ohri.ca/index.html).

Using decision aids to assist clinical management and counseling may represent a feasible, low-cost strategy to support patient decision-making in many scenarios. Clinicians may use or modify published decision aid tools to provide patients to use on their own, assist patient–provider communication, and guide counseling and intervention to support AYAs through the decision-making process.

Psychosocial Support

Some patients may need more comprehensive programs of support and individualized attention to address fertility-related questions, concerns, and counseling needs. Referral to trusted sources of information that may be easily accessed by patients is also needed for self-guided exploration of options surrounding fertility care, posttreatment fertility preservation, and planning for future family building, particularly in posttreatment survivorship. Exploration of the ways in which psychosocial and decision support interventions may be translated to the pediatric oncology setting is also needed. It has been shown that parental and patient concerns about fertility and future parenthood are often discordant, with parents and providers underestimating the degree of children's concern. Thus, clinicians treating underage minors should be careful when using parents' proxy reports and remember the limitations of parental awareness of children's concerns. Developmentally appropriate guidelines and resources to appropriately involve younger patients in fertility-related discussions need further development. Nevertheless, as previously suggested, providing opportunities for younger patients to be involved in conversations and to have a safe place to ask questions or express concerns is a key aspect of care.

Survivorship Care

Long-term AYA survivorship care plans often fail to provide follow-up fertility care after treatment. Survivors of childhood cancer may be more likely to receive fertility testing in accordance with surveillance guidelines set by the Children's Oncology Group. However, fertility-related knowledge among childhood cancer survivors is still poor and counseling is warranted beyond the mere testing of reproductive function. Likewise, regular fertility testing and monitoring among patients diagnosed within the AYA age range is often missing from survivorship care and should be offered whenever medically indicated aligned with survivors' parenthood goals and interest. These gaps in care prevent AYAs from accessing fertility-related care and psychosocial support when needed.

Posttreatment fertility preservation may be an option for women who were unable to preserve fertility before treatment but have a diminished ovarian reserve and are at risk for early menopause. Family building after cancer may require IVF, surrogacy, or adoption and can include medical, legal, financial, and/or logistical barriers that survivors should be aware of. Early planning and preparation to overcome these barriers may help survivors avoid or mitigate risks and challenges associated with alternative family-building options.

In posttreatment survivorship, undergoing an evaluation and first learning about fertility problems after cancer may initially increase patient distress but will also allow for early intervention if needed. For female patients, clinicians may need to be proactive in providing guidance even to those who may express disinterest or who do not feel ready to think about family building if there is reason to believe they may be at risk for premature ovarian failure. At younger ages and among females with heightened fertility distress, postponement and avoidance of fertility may be used to avoid or minimize distress. This may result in women missing their narrowed window of opportunity to have a biologically related child, if desired.

Clinicians may need to encourage patients to start thinking about their options for achieving parenthood early so that they understand the processes involved and potential barriers. Alternative family-building options include adoption, donor gametes, and/or surrogacy with a gestational carrier, and it is important to make sure patients are aware that having a biologically related child via pregnancy is not the only option to achieve parenthood. Alternative family-building options, however, are often associated with high costs and medical, legal, and/or logistical difficulties. It may be important to counsel patients that early planning will help to avoid or mitigate some difficulties, such as preparing financially for costs or understanding state-specific laws regulating surrogacy. Cancer survivors may also have a more difficult time adopting, particularly if they had a late-stage cancer, as discrimination by adoption agencies and birth parents has been reported.

Providing AYAs an opportunity to learn about reproductive options and family-building options also allows time for them to adjust psychologically to perceived bad news or disappointment associated with limited reproductive options, reframe expectations for how they might achieve parenthood, and make decisions about what they want for the future and plan ahead. Some survivors decide against having children following cancer treatment; in this case, normalizing decisions for a childless lifestyle is warranted.

The extent and nature of fertility concerns may differ between males and females, with some indication that females tend to be more distressed than males. Concerns may also differ by age. As women get older, anxieties about the metaphorical "racing biological clock" may arise, and greater reproductive concerns have been associated with depressive symptomatology and reduced quality of life.

Parents tend to underestimate levels of reproductive concern and importance of achieving parenthood in their adolescent daughters and sons, expecting them to prioritize survival. Similarly, AYAs have reported frustration and anger with clinical care teams who are perceived to communicate a message of "being happy with survival" and who fail to address posttreatment survivorship issues that are important to achieving life goals, including having children and building a family.

There may be social or interpersonal stressors related to fertility that are upsetting and difficult for patients and survivors to cope with. For example, AYAs may struggle watching friends or peers who are building their families, or couples may have difficulty communicating about fertility challenges and making decisions about family-building options. Addressing the psychosocial context within which fertility concerns exist is important for treating the whole patient and providing comprehensive care.

Cultural and Diversity Awareness

Clinicians should be mindful that AYA patients may come from diverse cultural backgrounds and may have different beliefs. Due to frequent assumptions about heterosexuality in the context of healthcare, it is important to be conscious of the unique needs of individuals based on self-identified gender and sexual identities, and to feel prepared to discuss such needs. Clinicians must be inclusive and respectful during clinical encounters and aware of the language they use, preconceived assumptions, and overall communication around gender and sexual orientation and cultural assumptions.

Sexual health and fertility counseling should be inclusive of AYAs who identify as gender and/or sexual minorities.

Whether discrimination is actual or perceived, gender-nonconforming and sexual minority youths report higher rates of feeling misunderstood and less satisfaction with care in oncology settings compared to heterosexual patients. Historically, AYAs identifying within gender/sexual minority groups also have lower rates of healthcare utilization, and thus are at greater risk for lacking basic medical care or counseling and having low knowledge of sexual and reproductive health issues. It is important for clinicians to stay apprised of evolving sexual identity and sexual experiences among their patients, and to take a comprehensive sexual history by asking neutral questions and creating an inclusive environment. Sexual behaviors should be normalized, not stigmatized, and providers should offer accurate information to LGBTQI patients who may have less access than gender-conforming or heterosexual peers. They should confirm that patients are seeking regular preventive care and cancer screening even when it is inconsistent with their gender identity, such as Pap tests for transgender men who have a uterus and cervix. As with all patients, protected sexual intercourse should be encouraged because of the possibility of transmitting HPV and other sexually transmitted diseases.

Sexual minority AYAs with cancer are just as interested in discussing options for fertility preservation and family building as heterosexual and gender-aligned patients. However, their views on relationships, parenthood, and family building may differ from those with heteronormative and culturally mainstream views, based on gender and sexual identity factors. Some studies suggest that LGBTQI patients may feel less distress about infertility and less concerned about fertility problems affecting dating and relationships compared to heterosexual patients and may feel more open to and accepting of having children who are not biologically related to them, or not becoming a parent at all. For some, not subscribing to heteronormative assumptions about how one becomes a parent may facilitate adjustment to cancer-related effects on fertility.

It is important for clinicians to be aware that patients may have varying viewpoints on acceptable or ideal ways for achieving parenthood and family building.

Information about dating, fertility risks, and family-building options is still valuable to LGBTQI patients and should be tailored to meet the unique needs of these subgroups and individuals. Tamargo et al. (2019) provide a comprehensive overview of the unique challenges LGBTQI patients may face related to fertility and fertility preservation, including barriers to healthcare due to concerns about confidentiality, need to disclose, and fear of discrimination.[11] Makadon et al. (2015) provide helpful guidelines for how to ask sexual health history questions during clinical encounters and "dos and don'ts" in taking a sexual history so as to provide an inclusive and affirming healthcare environment for LGBTQI patients.[12,13] See Chapter 3 for more on LGBT issues.

Professional Issues and Service Implementation

Recording and Communication

Depending on the care setting and facility, the extent of communication with other clinicians and members of a multidisciplinary team may vary, but communication is critical. Within teams, open communication and validation of

AYA patients' concerns and their lived experiences regarding their sexual and reproductive health are essential. All providers should be continuously made aware of potential reproductive and sexual health problems and concerns.

The following points provide a useful guide on communication and recording.

- An open and nonjudgmental attitude is emphasized.
- Given the sensitive nature of these topics and depending on the wishes of the patient, not all sensitive information should be shared with all providers and/or caregivers (see also the section "Legal Responsibilities" below).
- Whenever possible, review of medical charts or consulting with the treating oncology team can be helpful to determine treatment-specific side effects on sexual and reproductive health (e.g., gonadotoxicity, mutilation of reproductive organs, hormonal effects) so the clinician can provide more in-depth counseling to patients.
- Providers should be aware of their own personal biases (e.g., their own attitudes to sex and reproduction) and should make sure they do not stand in the way of their communication within teams and with patients.
- Care provided regarding sexual and reproductive health should always be noted in patients' medical records. However, the extent and detail of recorded information may vary. For example, some patients may not wish to have their sexual problems shared with the whole care team.
- In some cases, it may be important **not** to disclose the sexual orientation of patients; using generic pronouns and terms like "a partner" can facilitate this. With AYAs under the age of 18, it is important to clarify the legal obligation to share information with their legal guardians. This may hamper an open patient–provider relationship (also if patients are accompanied by their parents), and in such cases communication may not be so much about exploring the lived experiences of patients but rather providing educational material/information about reproductive and sexual health (see also the ethical dilemmas explored below).

Legal Responsibilities

Providing sexual and reproductive health counseling to AYAs can be difficult, but it is the provider's obligation to deliver holistic care and not neglect these topics. Guidelines recommend, for example, fertility counseling for any at-risk patient of reproductive age. Yet, in the case of AYAs, the need to discuss such issues has to be weighed against the patient's (cognitive) developmental level and sexual maturity. This extends beyond considering the legal age of 18; for instance, providers should consider whether patients are sexually experienced so as not to overwhelm or belittle them with unfit information.

A healthy attitude toward sexuality should be promoted. An emphasis on safer sex practices as well as sexual rights (e.g., the right to say no) for both partnered and unpartnered AYAs is important.

*Although rare, discussions about sexual health sometimes solicit the disclosure of sexual misuse or abuse, and emotional support as well as legal steps should be taken, **depending on each case**.*

If AYAs are in a relationship, their partners may be included in sexual and reproductive health counseling to facilitate and help manage procedures and potential side effects. However, if AYAs are partnered but not legally married or in a registered partnership, the (lacking) legal rights of a partner need to be discussed too. This becomes particularly important when considering fertility preservation. Partnered AYAs may be faced with the decision between freezing sperm/oocytes or embryos. This decision can be stressful for the patient (e.g., if doubting the current relationship) and should be discussed with great care, but it may also have legal implications.

Laws and regulations governing fertility preservation and ownership of cryopreserved material vary across countries (and within some countries) and must be reviewed with patients (and their partners) as a part of the informed consent process.

Married partners may have different rights over the possession of embryos than unmarried partners who produced embryos for the purposes of fertility preservation, and legal ownership and individual rights may change with divorce. Laws will also vary regulating the rights of legal guardians, who may or may not have legal ownership of cryopreserved material produced by underage children. Such rights may become even more complicated and emotionally laden if the AYA patient dies (e.g., interest of partner vs. parents of the deceased patient). For each clinical setting and country, the legal specifications need to be clarified and discussed within the care team and with patients.

Extrapolating from the example above, legal responsibilities become even more complex when treating underage minors, and the rights of parents and patients need to be discussed.

Clinicians should be cautious when using parent-proxy reports, given that parents may be unaware of their children's concerns.

Developmentally appropriate guidelines and resources to appropriately involve younger patients in sexual and fertility-related discussions need further development. Nevertheless, as previously suggested, providing opportunities for young patients to be involved in conversations and to have a safe place to ask questions or express concerns is a key aspect of care. Thereby, the legal obligation to disclose information to parents—if requested—needs to be clarified. Permission from parents should be obtained to also have sexual and reproductive health discussion without them present. See Box 4.5.

Ethical Dilemmas: Age and Maturity

As noted above, treating underage AYA patients can come with legal and development-specific considerations and dilemmas. Therefore, clinicians should:

> **Box 4.5 Privileging AYA Privacy and Confidentiality**
>
> Clinical judgment is needed to navigate parents' role and involvement, but it is recommended that all AYA patients have the opportunity to speak with their clinicians without parents present to allow privacy and confidentiality. When needed, clinicians may need to encourage parents to agree to private conversations between the clinician and underage patient to allow a safe space to ask questions and receive counseling.

- Assess the developmental stage of the AYA patient and defer counseling about sexual function until the patient reaches sexual maturity and/or expresses interest in sexual health/activity. Younger AYAs who have missed school due to illness may have also missed sex education classes and time to explore their sexuality together with peers. Thus, they may have lower levels of health and sexual knowledge than same-age peers.
- Obtain permission from parents to have sexual and reproductive health discussions without them present.
- Emphasize parents' beliefs, worries, and concerns too, given that they have to consent to any intervention (e.g., fertility preservation). An ethical dilemma could arise if an underage patient wants to opt for fertility preservation but the parents do not consent. In such cases, psychoeducation and communication between family members may be facilitated and decisional satisfaction emphasized.

The assessment of sexual and reproductive health of AYA survivors should be embedded in a broader perspective that also takes sociocultural and religious factors into account. In general, cultural and social norms that dissuade help seeking around sensitive topics like sexuality and fertility will affect access to care. Research that focused on the role of sociocultural and religious factors in AYA cancer patients is limited. Studies often use race and ethnicity as markers of cultural differences and conflate the effect of these factors with socioeconomic status.

Common factors that should be considered are:

- Language barriers and limited financial resources affect patients' access to care and ability to express concerns and communicate with the medical team. Patience, adjusting the language used, and/or use of certified translators may be warranted.
- In many cultures, sexual topics are considered taboo and cause embarrassment or shame, which may further prevent patients from initiating discussions with clinicians and seeking medical care and support.
- Cultural stereotypes about masculinity and femininity can exacerbate difficulties related to identity reformation after cancer and acceptance of body changes, especially at a young age.
- Social norms and gender stereotypes vary across cultures and religions, and the cultural acceptability of expressing sexual/reproductive problems and willingness to seek help differ. Sexual dysfunction and infertility can challenge commonly held beliefs and definitions of manhood and womanhood,

especially if patients are young. Fertility problems may challenge traditional expectations about how fatherhood and motherhood can be achieved after cancer at a young age. Thus, AYAs' attitudes and potential difficulties/concerns need to be assessed and addressed in an open-minded manner.

- The importance of having children and expectations for achieving fatherhood/motherhood vary across cultures and individuals. These may shape perceptions about the importance of being biologically related to a child or views on reproductive medicine, including the use of embryos to conceive. Such attitudes may present barriers to communication and care and should be explored.

Ethical Dilemmas: Managing Patient Expectations

While care providers typically try to act in the best interests of the patient, sometimes it is difficult to provide hope versus worst-case scenarios when trying to give a realistic picture. For example, potential (future) sexual problems should not be brushed off in the hope that they will not occur. Similarly, estimating potential infertility risk and/or outcomes of fertility preservation requires careful communication and the management of realistic hope. Too often, fertility preservation is presented to patients as a reassurance/backup plan, but whether assisted reproductive technologies will work for each patient in the future is questionable. Thus, careful communication, consultation with other experts, and honesty need to be emphasized.

Policy, Training, Supervision

Policies for discussions and referrals for appropriate patients should be in place but may vary greatly depending on the clinical setting, facility, and resources. However, minimal standards, such as initiating discussions with patients, educating them about sexual and reproductive health, and offering appropriate referrals, should be met. See Box 4.6.

Some interventions have been developed to prepare providers for having such clinical discussions with patients. Recently, a short educational intervention, Fex-Can, was developed to overcome patient–provider barriers to communicating about sexuality and fertility in oncology.[14] The intervention targets nurses and was shown to improve clinical care by increasing their understanding of patients' sex- and fertility-related needs and overcoming barriers to having appropriate discussions. A more in-depth program is ENRICH (Educating Nurses about Reproductive Issues in Cancer Healthcare), an

Box 4.6 Ethical Oversight and Training/Supervision

There may be dedicated staff/confidants who can be approached and consulted should ethical uncertainties or dilemmas arise. Team discussions may also be helpful. Continuous training, minimum-standard policies, and supervision (e.g., by NPs, sexologists, psychologists, reproductive endocrinologists) will help raise awareness of sexual and reproductive issues among AYAs. All of the above is vital to offering appropriate care and equal opportunities to all patients, irrespective of their providers.

online training program for oncology nurses to promote communication about reproductive health (e.g., infertility risk, fertility preservation, sexual health) with AYA patients.[15] The online course includes eight modules about reproductive health, family-building options, sexual health, communication, and practical applications and has been shown to improve nurses' knowledge and communication skills.

The ECHO intervention (Enriching Communication for Health Professionals in Oncofertility) was developed based on the ENRICH program as an online training program for not only nurses but also allied health clinicians. including physician assistants, social workers, and psychologists. to improve their knowledge and communication about reproductive health with AYA patients. In sum, continuous training, policies, and ongoing supervision can help clinicians to appropriately address young patients' concerns and deal with certain dilemmas and problems.

Open, nonjudgmental communication with patients, with caregivers, and within the clinical care team is to be emphasized at all times.

References

1. Coccia PF, Pappo AS, Beaupin L, et al. Adolescent and young adult oncology, version 2.2018, NCCN clinical practice guidelines in oncology. *J Nat Compr Cancer Netw* 2018;16(1):66–97. doi:10.6004/jnccn.2018.0001

2. Wettergren L, Kent EE, Mitchell SA, et al. Cancer negatively impacts on sexual function in adolescents and young adults: the AYA HOPE study. *Psychooncology* 2017;26(10):1632–1639. doi:10.1002/pon.4181

3. Bober SL, Zhou ES, Chen B, et al. Sexual function in childhood cancer survivors: a report from Project REACH. *J Sex Med* 2013;10(8):2084–2093. doi:10.1111/jsm.12193

4. Coccia PF. Overview of adolescent and young adult oncology. *J Oncol Pract* 2019;15(5):235–237. doi:10.1200/JOP.19.00075

5. Sodergren SC, Husson O, Robinson J, et al. Systematic review of the health-related quality of life issues facing adolescents and young adults with cancer. *Qual Life Res* 2017;26(7):1659–1672. doi:10.1007/s11136-017-1520-x

6. Bober SL, Reese JB, Barbera L, et al. How to ask and what to do: a guide for clinical inquiry and intervention regarding female sexual health after cancer. *Curr Opin Support Palliat Care* 2016;10(1):44–54. doi:10.1097/SPC.0000000000000186

7. Kemertzis M, Ranjithakumaran H, Hand M, et al. Fertility preservation toolkit: a clinician resource to assist clinical discussion and decision making in pediatric and adolescent oncology. *J Pediatr Hematol Oncol* 2018;40(3):e133–139. doi:10.1097/MPH.0000000000001103

8. Aubin S, Perez S. The clinician's toolbox: assessing the sexual impacts of cancer on adolescents and young adults with cancer (AYAC). *Sex Med* 2015;3(3):198–212. doi:10.1002/sm2.75

9. Suckling JA, Kennedy R, Lethaby A, Roberts H. Local oestrogen for vaginal atrophy in postmenopausal women. *Cochrane Database Syst Rev* 2006. doi:10.1002/14651858.CD001500.pub2

10. Diaz-Garcia C, Domingo J, Garcia-Velasco JA, et al. Oocyte vitrification versus ovarian cortex transplantation in fertility preservation for adult women undergoing gonadotoxic treatments: a prospective cohort study. *Fertil Steril* 2018;109(3):478–485. doi:10.1016/j.fertnstert.2017.11.018

11. Tamargo C, Quinn G, Schabath MB, Vadaparampil ST. The importance of disclosure for sexual minorities in oncofertility cases. In: Woodruff TK, Gosiengfiao YC, eds. *Pediatric and Adolescent Oncofertility: Best Practices and Emerging Technologies.* Cham: Springer International Publishing; 2017:193–207. doi:10.1007/978-3-319-32973-4_13

12. Makadon HJ, Goldhammer H. Taking a sexual history and creating affirming environments for lesbian, gay, bisexual, and transgender people. *J Miss State Med Assoc* 2015;56(12):358–362.

13. Hadland SE, Yehia BR, Makadon HJ. Caring for lesbian, gay, bisexual, transgender, and questioning youth in inclusive and affirmative environments. *Pediatr Clin North Am* 2016;63(6):955–969. doi:10.1016/j.pcl.2016.07.001

14. Lampic C, Ljungman L, Micaux Obol C, et al. A web-based psycho-educational intervention (Fex-Can) targeting sexual dysfunction and fertility-related distress in young adults with cancer: study protocol of a randomized controlled trial. *BMC Cancer* 2019;19(1):344. doi:10.1186/s12885-019-5518-3

15. Vadaparampil ST, Gwede CK, Meade C, et al. ENRICH: a promising oncology nurse training program to implement ASCO clinical practice guidelines on fertility for AYA cancer patients. *Patient Educ Couns* 2016;99(11):1907–1910. doi:10.1016/j.pec.2016.05.013

Further Reading

Sexual Health

Aubin S, Perez S. The clinician's toolbox: assessing the sexual impacts of cancer on adolescents and young adults with cancer (AYAC). *Sex Med* 2015;3(3):198–212.

This article provides a comprehensive guide to assessing sexual function in AYAs, including interview questions, need for review of medical records, and self-report measures of functioning. Resources that may be distributed to patients are included.

Bober SL, Reese JB, Barbera L, et al. How to ask and what to do: a guide for clinical inquiry and intervention regarding female sexual health after cancer. *Curr Opin Support Palliat Care* 2016;10(1):44–54.

This study provides a model of clinical inquiry tailored to female survivors of cancer who report sexual dysfunction after treatment. It offers resources describing symptoms and treatments that may be distributed directly to patients as well as a questionnaire measure of overall sexual function.

Park ER, Norris RL, Bober SL. Sexual health communication during cancer care: barriers and recommendations. *Cancer J* 2009;15(1):74–77.

Reviews an adaptive behavioral health counseling model as a framework for sexual health communication with cancer patients in multidisciplinary settings. It based on the 5 A's model: Ask, Advise, Assess, Assist, and Arrange Follow-up.

Wettergren L, Kent EE, Mitchell SA, et al. Cancer negatively impacts on sexual function in adolescents and young adults: the AYA HOPE study. *Psychooncology* 2017;26(10):1632–1639.

In this longitudinal survey study, the AYA HOPE Study Collaborative Group investigated sexual functioning in a large cohort (n = 465) of AYA survivors of cancer. Findings include the prevalence, impact, and duration of sexual side effects of cancer treatment up to 2 years after diagnosis.

Reproductive Health

Anazodo A, Laws P, Logan S, et al. How can we improve oncofertility care for patients? A systematic scoping review of current international practice and models of care. *Hum Reprod Update* 2019;25(2):159–179.

This systematic review covers the components of onco-fertility care as defined by patients and clinicians, as well as the barriers, facilitators, and challenges of onco-fertility models of care and real-world application of guidelines.

Kemertzis M, Ranjithakumaran H, Hand M, et al. Fertility preservation toolkit: a clinician resource to assist clinical discussion and decision making in pediatric and adolescent oncology. *J Pediatr Hematol Oncol* 2018;40(3):e133–e139.

This article describes the development of a clinician resource for onco-fertility care including a description of items needed to support fertility-preservation counseling and referral.

Quinn GP, Vadaparampil ST, ed. *Reproductive Health and Cancer in Adolescents and Young Adults.* The Netherlands: Springer, 2012.

This book reviews the needs of male and female patients related to onco-fertility care, describes effective communication strategies and proactive measures for healthcare professionals to use, and discusses gaps in the literature where more research is needed. Topics include fertility preservation, pregnancy and cancer, nontraditional family building, counseling in pediatric settings, and legal and ethical issues, among others, as well as sexual health topics related to contraceptive counseling and sexual health during treatment.

Woodruff TK, Clayman ML, Waimey KE, eds. *Oncofertility Communication: Sharing Information and Building Relationships Across Disciplines.* New York: Springer-Verlag, 2014.

This book describes onco-fertility issues that relate to the role of healthcare professionals across disciplines, including oncology, reproductive medicine, psychosocial work, and genetics. The book discusses a range of topics related to multidisciplinary onco-fertility care, including communication and counseling across patient groups such as high-risk patients and in pediatric settings, supporting patients' decision-making, genetic counseling, and incorporating insurance education into the fertility-preservation process.

Adapted with permission from:

Benedict C, Thom B, Teplinsky E, Carleton J, Kelvin JF. Family-building after breast cancer: considering the effect on adherence to adjuvant endocrine therapy. *Clin Breast Cancer* 2017;17(3):165–170.

Chapter 5

Principles of Treatment of Sexual Dysfunction

Michelle Peate and Ilona Juraskova

Learning Objectives

After reading this chapter the clinician will be able to:

1. Identify the impact of cancer treatment on psychosexual well-being (e.g., body image and sexual dysfunction/problems) in males and females
2. Assess the potential needs of patients for addressing psychosexual problems, with specific knowledge of differences according to cancer site and individual factors
3. Identify and provide access to effective evidence-based interventions for sexual dysfunction/problems

Background Evidence

The prevalence of cancer-related sexual dysfunction and body image problems varies according to diagnosis and treatment, affecting at least half of those treated for pelvic malignancies or breast cancers (with some reports citing over 90%) and greater than a quarter of patients with other cancers.[1–4] These rates are higher than what is seen in the general population.[5] Sexual dysfunction is associated with psychosocial morbidities such as depression and poorer self-assessed general health, lower relationship satisfaction, psychosocial adjustment problems, and diminished quality of life in the longer term.[2,5–7] It can also impact intimate relationships and identity.[2] Posttreatment effects can result in poorer body image and satisfaction, feelings of being unattractive, shame, guilt, avoidance, fear, and anxiety.[2] This creates a cycle of increasing morbidity that further impairs sexual functioning.[2] Sexual issues are consistently reported as a significant unmet need by cancer patients.[8]

The disruption to sexual well-being in cancer patients can occur across the phases of the sexual response cycle—arousal, plateau, orgasm, and resolution—and can be affected by both physical symptoms (e.g., changes in physiologic structure, vaginal dryness, dyspareunia, and erectile dysfunction) and psychological factors (e.g., body image, low self-esteem, reduced desire and arousal, and distress).[2,3]

The type of cancer treatment that the patient receives is a key factor in physical symptoms that often result in sexual dysfunction (Table 5.1).[1,2]

Table 5.1 Sexual Consequences of Cancer Treatments

Treatment	Impact on Sexual Function In Women	In Men
Surgery	*Pelvic surgeries* can result in structural alterations, local nerve damage, and changes in vascularization, which affect sexual response. *Colorectal surgeries* can result in physiologic changes that result in soiling, incontinence, and pain. *Bladder surgeries* can result in damage to the nerves that result in lubrication and sexual response. *Breast surgeries* can result in scarring, pain, lost breast and nipple sensation. *Brain surgeries* (right hemisphere) can impact arousal and orgasm. *Face and neck surgical changes* can interfere with partner interactions (e.g., kissing and oral sex). Disfigurement as a result of surgery can have an impact on body image and result in distress.[2]	*Pelvic surgery* can result in nerve damage and vascular changes that lead to erectile dysfunction.[1] The majority of men undergoing *radical prostatectomy* (RP) never regain pretreatment levels of erectile function[23] and will find that erectile dysfunction is immediately apparent after treatment. Posttreatment orgasmic dysfunctions, as well as climacturia, are also common in men treated with RP. These dysfunctions can cause many men psychological distress and, in turn, become associated with a reduction in quality of life, loss of self-esteem, and relationship difficulties. Penile length loss, another commonly reported side effect of RP, causes patients significant distress. It is thought that penile shortening is caused by neural damage, if not directly, then at least indirectly through erectile dysfunction; however, the mechanism is unknown.[24]
Radiotherapy	Radiotherapy and brachytherapy in general are associated with fatigue and poorer body image. Other effects are related to the region it is applied: - *Pelvic area:* vaginal stenosis, shortening, incontinence, vasoconstriction, lymphedema, and loss of genital sensitivity - *Anal area:* urgency - *Breast area:* scarring, burns, lymphedema, skin thickening - *Total body irradiation* can contribute to genital tissue sensitivity, atrophy, or scarring. Impact of radiotherapy persists for several years.[2]	External-beam radiation therapy and brachytherapy in the *pelvic area* can directly damage tissues and nerves necessary for a strong erection, resulting in erectile dysfunction.[1] These men are likely to experience a progressive decline in sexual functioning over a long period, caused by the process of ionizing radiation, which accelerates the microvascular angiopathic changes, thus causing cavernosal fibrosis and endothelial dysfunction. *Total body irradiation* can contribute to genital tissue sensitivity, atrophy, or scarring.[25]

(continued)

Table 5.1 Continued

Treatment	Impact on Sexual Function In Women	In Men
Chemotherapy	Some chemotherapies (e.g., those with alkylating agents) are cytotoxic to the ovaries and can result in premature ovarian failure (i.e., menopause) by depleting the ovarian follicle pool. The broader impacts of chemotherapy such as fatigue, vaginal or rectal mucosal toxicity, alopecia, weight changes, and gastrointestinal issues can interfere with sexuality, desire, and arousal.[2]	Some side effects of chemotherapy in men include hair loss, mouth sores, nausea and vomiting, diarrhea, loss of appetite, infections, easy bruising, and fatigue. These side effects often have an indirect effect on sexual functioning through desire, arousal, and body image.
Endocrine (hormonal) therapy	Endocrine therapy causes estrogen depletion, which essentially results in menopausal symptoms such as vaginal dryness and vulvovaginal atrophy.[2] Dryness predicts low desire, dyspareunia, decreased satisfaction, and poor sexual function.[3]	Hormonal treatments can damage the nerves and blood supply, resulting in erection problems. Hormonal changes secondary to androgen deprivation therapy can also result in erectile dysfunction.[1]
Hematopoietic stem cell transplantation	Allogenic bone marrow transplantation is associated with graft-versus-host disease (GVHD), which can have systemic or local effects—GVHD in the genital and mucous membranes. Symptoms such as dryness, stenosis, itching, scarring, and structural changes, accompanied by dyspareunia and loss of desire, have a severe impact on sexual functioning.[2] High-dose corticosteroids are a common component of chronic GVHD treatment and have major impacts on body image and mental health.[25]	Chronic GVHD can also cause inflammation, rash, and sensitivity in the skin of the penis.[25] High-dose corticosteroids are a common component of chronic GVHD treatment and have major impacts on body image and mental health.[25]

Education about the potential effect of cancer treatments on sexual function should be part of the informed consent process to treatment, as well as any dialogue around plans for symptom and side effect management where the chosen therapies may affect sexual function.[9] Evidence demonstrates that patients who recall having had a conversation with a clinician about sexual issues experience reduced sexual morbidity (by almost threefold).[5]

Presenting Problems

The impact of cancer treatment can affect all phases of the human sexual response cycle (Figure 5.1):

- *Desire phase:* The ability to feel desire, and that others might desire them sexually, can be affected by body image and sexuality changes, depression, fatigue, and treatment side effects (e.g., nausea, diarrhea, mucositis).
- *Arousal phase:* In women, loss of vaginal lubrication and changes to the vagina (i.e., shortening or narrowing) can lead to pain and reduce their ability to relax and enjoy arousal. In men, the ability to get and keep an erection can be affected by testosterone changes, nerve injury, scarring and fibrosis, and others.
- *Orgasm:* Some women may be unable to reach the threshold necessary to have an orgasm, or if orgasm is achieved, it may be less intense and less enjoyable. In men, problems with orgasm may be a failure to ejaculate or retrograde ejaculation. This may be a result of anxiety and depression, a side effect of drugs used in treatment, or a result of nerve damage (in the case of ejaculation). Climacturia (orgasm-associated urinary incontinence), decreased orgasm intensity, lack of orgasm, and pain during orgasm are also common in men after treatment.

The linear model of the human sexual response cycle, originally proposed by has served as the paradigm for sexual functioning. In 2002, Basson proposed a model of sexual response that is circular and more complex than the traditional linear model to better capture women's sexual responses, particularly those who are in long-term relationships.[10] This nonlinear model of sexual response incorporates the need for intimacy and recognizes that desire can be responsive or spontaneous, desire may come either before or

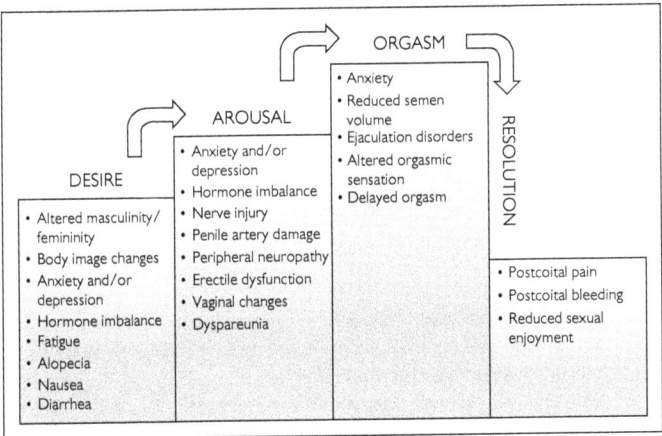

Figure 5.1 Factors affecting the human sexual response cycle

Adapted from White (2013)[17]

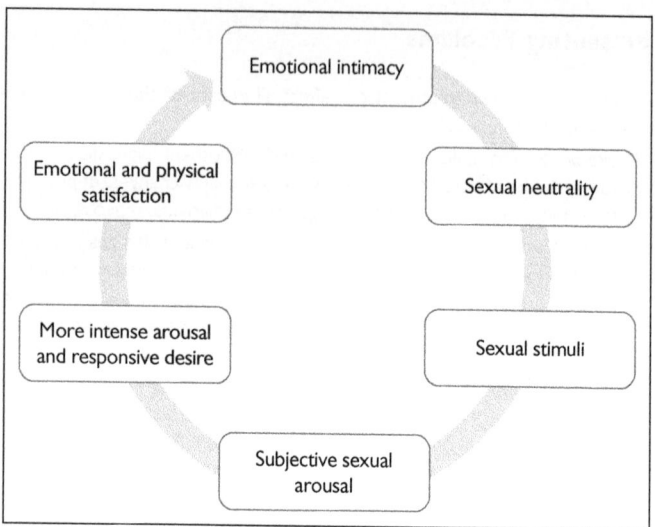

Figure 5.2 Basson's model of sexual response
Based on Basson (2002)[10]

after arousal, orgasm may contribute to but is not necessary for satisfaction, relationship factors impact the cycle as costs or rewards and affect one's willingness and ability to participate in sex, and one can enter the cycle at several points. This has been a paradigm shift in the understanding and conceptualization of a "normal" sexual response—in other words, the distinction between certain phases (e.g., desire and arousal) may be artificial and the process is not always linear (Figure 5.2). The fifth edition of the American Psychiatric Association's *Diagnostic and Statistical Manual of Mental Disorders* (DSM-5) has added gender-specific sexual dysfunctions, and, for females, sexual desire and arousal disorders have been combined into one disorder: female sexual interest/arousal disorder.

When dealing with sexual dysfunction in cancer patients,

⚠ Discussions and interventions should be congruent with the patient's literacy level, cultural/religious beliefs, partner status, age, sexual orientation, and cancer stage:

1. **Literacy**—Patients with poor literacy have an array of difficulties with written and oral communication that may limit their understanding of cancer treatments and related side effects.
2. **Culture**—Cultural background and varying degrees of comfort regarding discussion of sexual health concerns have been found to impact the likelihood that clinicians will engage in communication with patients.[11]

3. **Partner status**—The misperception that sexual well-being is irrelevant for certain survivors (e.g., unpartnered) is a common barrier to discussion (see also Chapter 3 for details relating to LGBTQ+ patients).[12]
4. **Sexuality**—Making assumptions about "normal" sexuality on the basis of sexual orientation results in the neglect of the needs of significant numbers of LGBTQ+ individuals (see Chapter 3 for more details).[13]
5. **Age**—Assumptions about the sexuality of older patients frequently prevent the initiation of discussions about sexual health issues.[14] Sexuality is relevant to people at any age.
6. **Palliative care**—Although palliative care patients and their partners want to discuss sexual functioning and intimacy, these conversations are uncommon.[15] Sexuality continues to be important at the end of life.

Investigations for Key Differential Diagnoses

Discussing the sexual consequences of cancer can be challenging and appears to occur more often with male than female patients.[16] The core driver for intervention commonly relates to patients' dissatisfaction with their sexual life (sexual inactivity in itself is not problematic) and/or distress or avoidance as a result of sexual difficulties, as well as availability of interventions. Psychosocial and/or psychosexual counseling should be offered to all patients with cancer with the goal of improving sexual response, body image, self-esteem, intimacy and relationship issues, and overall sexual functioning and satisfaction.

Clinicians should proactively ask if the patient has noticed any changes in sexual interest, arousal, sexual pain, or orgasmic and ejaculatory experience. A sample question to ask is, "Many patients in a similar situation as you have fears or worries about what it might feel like to resume sexual life again. Is that something that is worrying you?"[17] The American Society of Clinical Oncology (ASCO; https://ascopubs.org/doi/full/10.1200/JCO.2017.75.8995) recommends the following:

- The topic of sexual function should be discussed with the patient alone, with the option of later partner inclusion if desired by the patient.[9]
- This discussion should be initiated at the time of diagnosis and continued periodically at varied points of treatment and survivorship to assess or address any changes.

Routine use of patient-reported outcome measures may help identify patients and survivors with sexual problems:

- As a primary screening tool, the National Comprehensive Cancer Network (NCCN) recommends the Brief Sexual Symptom Checklist for Women (http://www.aftercancer.co/wp-content/uploads/2015/11/NCCN-Symptom-Femal.pdf).

- Another self-assessment option is a single-item screener published by the Patient-Reported Outcomes Measurement Information System (PROMIS) group and the Scientific Network on Female Sexual Health and Cancer (https://www.ncbi.nlm.nih.gov/pmc/articles/PMC4579234/).
- More in-depth assessment in women can be achieved by using the PROMIS Sexual Function and Satisfaction measures (http://www.healthmeasures.net/images/PROMIS/manuals/PROMIS_Sexual_Function_and_Satisfaction_Measures_User_Manual_v1.0_and_v2.0.pdf) and the Female Sexual Function Index (FSFI https://www.fsfiquestionnaire.com/), both of which have been validated in cancer patients.
- In men, the International Index of Erectile Function (IIEF; https://www.baus.org.uk/_userfiles/pages/files/Patients/Leaflets/iief.pdf) is recommended as a comprehensive assessment tool.
- Many of the existing European Organisation for Research and Treatment of Cancer (EORTC) quality-of-life instruments also include a few questions on sexual function. A new 22-item Sexual Health Questionnaire (the EORTC SHQ-22) is in its final stages of psychometric evaluation.[18]

Clinical Management

Generally, gentle sexual activity following cancer treatment is safe. There are a number of physical and pharmacologic interventions that can assist, and typically a multifaceted, biopsychosocial approach is needed.[2] For example, should a woman present with pain and dryness, the management might include a combination of moisturizers and lubricants, vaginal dilator therapy, pelvic floor physiotherapy, and/or topical analgesia, combined with education and/or psychological or psychosexual therapy. Although erectile dysfunction is often managed pharmacologically, a holistic approach to care is recommended. Box 5.1 lists precipitating and maintaining factors for sexual dysfunction.

Box 5.1 Precipitating and Maintaining Factors for Sexual Difficulties

Difficulties in sexual functioning appear to be highly prevalent in patients/survivors experiencing the following precipitating and maintaining factors:[1,3,7]
- Body image disturbance and adjustment, low self-esteem, altered femininity or masculinity
- Sexual dissatisfaction, relationship dissatisfaction, infertility concerns
- Vaginal dryness and dyspareunia, erectile and ejaculatory dysfunction
- Treatment-induced vasomotor symptoms, changes in genitalia
- Anxiety and depression
- Comorbidities and current medication should also be considered along with the likelihood of nerve/vascular integrity.

Stepped Approach to the Management of Sexual Dysfunction

White[17] recommends a stepped management approach:

1. **Communication:** Identify the problem (involving the partner where appropriate), helping the patient to communicate challenges and anxieties.
2. **Drug therapy:** Consider phosphodiesterase type 5 inhibitors (e.g., sildenafil [Viagra], tadalafil [Cialis], vardenafil [Levitra]) for erectile dysfunction or hormone replacement therapy for someone with testosterone deficiency or treatment-induced menopause, if medically safe. Nonpharmacologic options should be the initial treatment for most women, since current pharmacologic therapies for female sexual dysfunction have limited efficacy and are associated with side effects and risks.
3. **Mildly invasive management:** For women who have undergone pelvic radiotherapy or pelvic surgery, particularly those with vaginal reconstruction, and who experience treatment-induced vaginal changes, consider using vaginal dilator therapy; lubricants, vaginal moisturizers, or topical estrogens; and pelvic floor muscle relaxation exercises. For men, penile injections are recommended for erectile dysfunction not responding to oral therapy.
4. **Mechanical options:** Mechanical options include vacuum pumps and constriction rings for erectile dysfunction, vibrators (vaginal or clitoral) for orgasmic difficulties, a vaginal prosthesis for women without a vagina who want to have penetrative sex, or a penile prosthesis ("strap-on") for men who cannot maintain an erection.
5. **Surgical interventions:** Surgical interventions can include vaginal reconstruction or penile implants.

Psychological support (psychotherapy, sexual counseling, psychosexual therapy) is recommended throughout the assessment and management of sexual difficulties.

Biomedical Interventions

Describing biomedical interventions is beyond the scope of this chapter. For biomedical management, referrals to pelvic floor physiotherapists, urologists, endocrinologists, and/or sexual health specialists in consultation with the medical oncologist are recommended. Where available, specialist survivorship, sexual medicine, or menopause after cancer clinics may have established referral pathways. Psychosocial interventions for sexual dysfunction/difficulties need to accompany biomedical interventions.

Psychosocial Interventions

Psychosocial interventions may be appropriate for patients who experience anxiety or low mood, altered body image or sexuality, changes in sexual desire, or relationship or intimacy difficulties. There is growing evidence for the role of psychosocial interventions in managing sexual dysfunction (although stronger evidence from randomized controlled trials is still needed). For some patients, if biomedical and psychosocial interventions do not improve dysfunction, distress and avoidance of sexual intimacy can occur, followed by disconnection from a meaningful sexual relationship. This is where psychological and psychosexual therapy can help by facilitating sexual adjustment to the "new normal."

For women who are experiencing problems with general sexual response (desire, arousal, or orgasm), ASCO clinical guidelines recommend psychosocial and/or psychosexual counseling aiming to improve elements of sexual response and regular stimulation (including masturbation).[9] If specific issues that result in problems in sexual response are identified (e.g., body image), these can be addressed using the psychosocial interventions outlined in Table 5.2.[9]

In men who are experiencing erectile dysfunction, as described earlier in the chapter, the typical first-line treatment is pharmacologic, followed by mechanical or surgical interventions. ASCO guidelines also recommend psychosocial (couples) counseling alongside biomedical treatments with the goal of greater adaptation toward long-term use of treatments and regular stimulation (including masturbation).[9] If specific issues that result in problems in sexual response are identified, these can be addressed using the psychosocial interventions in Table 5.3.[9]

Table 5.2 Management of Key Issues for Women

Presenting Issue	Recommended Management/Interventions
Body image	Psychosocial counseling and couples-based interventions
Intimacy/relationships	Psychosocial counseling and couples-based interventions
Overall sexual functioning and satisfaction	Individual, couple, or group psychosocial counseling (in combination with physical exercise or pelvic floor physiotherapy where appropriate)
	Education and symptom management based on the patient's diagnosis
	Mental health counseling (for those with continued distress)
Vasomotor symptoms	Although the most effective intervention is hormone therapy, some women may be unwilling (contraindicated) or unable to take hormone therapy. *Pharmacologic alternatives* include selective serotonin reuptake inhibitors (SSRIs); however, these need to be carefully considered for potential interactions with cancer treatment. Paroxetine, sertraline, and fluoxetine (2D6 metabolism) should not be offered to women with breast cancer taking tamoxifen.
	Nonpharmacologic alternatives include cognitive-behavioral therapy (CBT) and/or clinical hypnosis. Other integrative therapies (e.g., acupuncture and slow breathing) may also help, but the evidence is less clear.
Genital symptoms (e.g., vaginal and/or vulval atrophy)	This symptom should be mainly managed through biomedical intervention (lubricants and moisturizers, low-dose estrogen, pelvic floor physiotherapy, and/or pain relief). However, in cases where genital symptoms affect intimacy, counseling may help. CBT and pelvic floor (Kegel) exercises may be useful to decrease anxiety and discomfort and can lower urinary tract symptoms.
Mental health (e.g., depression)	CBT

When treating male patients for sexual dysfunction/difficulties, there is a tendency to focus on restoration of erection-dependent sexual practices, with the use of medications, injections, vacuum devices, or implants. Yet these biomedical aids are not always effective or may be unappealing, and most couples stop using rehabilitation aids within the first 2 years.[19] It is important to promote sexual intimacy (i.e. erection-independent sexual activities and relational intimacy and physical affection; Figure 5.3) despite the many functional challenges these men experience.[19]

Aside from these general recommendations, the question is whether any specific psychosocial or psychosexual intervention is superior to another. For practical, easy-to-follow evidence-based treatment guides for the most common female and male sexual disorders seen in clinical practice, clinicians can consult two resources by Rowland.[20,21]

Table 5.3 Management of Key Issues for Men

Presenting Issue	Recommended Management
Body image	Psychosocial counseling covering issues such as weight changes, disfigurement, scarring, and hair loss
Intimacy/relationships	Individual or couples counseling
Overall sexual functioning and satisfaction	Psychosocial counseling and couples intervention in combination with erectile agents and devices
	Education on the changes in erection and alternative ways to maintain sexual intimacy
	Testosterone replacement therapy (when safe and indicated) is being recommended as the first-line treatment to alleviate hypoactive sexual desire disorder.
Vasomotor symptoms	Medical intervention is recommended. However, other integrative medicine options, such as acupuncture, slow-breathing techniques, and hypnosis (with evidence in women), may provide benefit. Psychosocial counseling (cognitive-behavioral therapy [CBT]) may provide benefit and reduce vasomotor symptoms and should be offered.
Genital symptoms	Mechanical intervention (i.e., vacuum erectile device [VED]) and/or medication is recommended. Phosphodiesterase type 5 inhibitors are the first-line treatment for erectile dysfunction. For men who don't respond to these medications, intracavernosal penile injections should be recommended. Alternatively, VEDs have been reported to restore erectile functioning. For patients who are not responding to these interventions, report adverse side effects, or want a permanent solution, surgical interventions such as a penile prosthesis are safe and efficacious.
	Treatment for climacturia includes the use of condoms during intercourse, pelvic floor rehabilitation, and bladder emptying and avoidance of fluid intake before sexual activity.
	Treatment for penis length loss includes VEDs or phosphodiesterase inhibitors.
Mental health (e.g., depression)	CBT

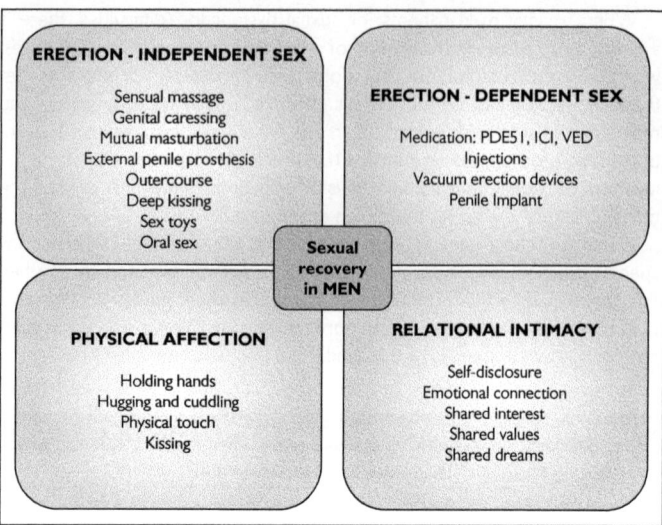

Figure 5.3 Approaches to sexual rehabilitation
Based on Walker et al. (2015)[18]

⚠ Special Considerations

- *Safety of sexual activity while immunosuppressed or with a significantly low thrombocyte count.* To reduce the risk of sexually transmitted infections, patients should use barrier contraceptives. Anal penetration is not advised due to increased risk of infection.
- *Avoiding unplanned pregnancy.* It is often recommended that patients avoid pregnancy for some months after completion of cancer treatment. Thus, patients should use contraceptives if engaging in sexual activity when normal fertility levels are reestablished.
- *Concerns about excess bleeding associated with chemotherapy-induced thrombocytopenia.* Using lubricants can help to reduce friction, along with gentle penetration. Anal penetration is not advised due to the increased risk of mucosal damage and bleeding.
- *Fear of "contamination" from radiotherapy or chemotherapy.* Some patients may raise concerns about passing on the radiation to their partner. There is no evidence to suggest that external-beam radiotherapy or byproducts of chemotherapy are transmissible. However, sexual contact should be avoided with patients treated with sealed or unsealed sources (e.g., iodine-131), who may still be considered radioactive.
- Close liaison with oncology colleagues by psychosexual practitioners is advised when psychological intervention programs are being discussed with patients and partners. A multidisciplinary approach is recommended when different treatments are under consideration.

Case Study: Painful Intercourse

Jane is a 45-year-old woman with a history of early stage breast cancer (treated with surgery, chemotherapy, and endocrine therapy) who was referred to the Menopause after Cancer Clinic for evaluation of symptoms, including sexual dysfunction. She reported that she experienced pain with penetration following her cancer treatment and, because of this, she has abstained from intercourse for the last 12 months. Abstinence means that she is not in pain (though she is experiencing vaginal dryness). However, she is concerned about the impact of this on her relationship with her husband—she is anxious that, in not meeting his sexual needs, he will leave her. Prior to her diagnosis, she reports that they had a very fulfilling sex life. Her desire is lower than she remembers. Her medical record did not indicate (as part of the regular screening process in this clinic) elevated depressive symptoms. She is not taking any other medications and her social history is otherwise unrevealing. She has not tried any interventions.

After working through the investigation process as described above, it was identified that in addition to lower desire, body image was also an issue for Jane. Individual and couples-based therapy was recommended to address body image concerns and relationship and intimacy issues (including suggestions for alternatives to penetrative sex). Jane was also referred to the Pelvic Pain Clinic for biomedical management (lubricants and moisturizers, pelvic floor physiotherapy, and/or pain relief) of her physical symptoms. With this multidisciplinary, collaborative approach, Jane was able to resume an intimate relationship with her husband.

Case Study: Erectile Dysfunction

Peter is a 60-year-old man with a history of prostate cancer (treated with a radical prostatectomy) who presented with erectile dysfunction. He had a noticed a lack of desire (compared with before cancer), and when he attempted to have sex or to masturbate, he had problems achieving an erection. He was not currently in a relationship. In addition to the recommended investigations above, because his affect was low he was asked to complete depression, anxiety, and stress scales, which indicated that he was clinically depressed. Cognitive-behavioral therapy (CBT) was recommended for the management of his depression, and he was referred to a urologist for pharmacologic (phosphodiesterase type 5 inhibitor or penile injection therapy) and/or mechanical (vacuum erectile device) management of the erectile dysfunction. His treatment plan also included psychosocial counseling and resource provision about desire and self-pleasure. The CBT helped Peter's mood, and he reported an increase in desire. Pharmacologic management helped him to achieve erections and resume a degree of pleasure. The ability to achieve erections also helped with his confidence.

Professional Issues and Service Implementation

Recording and Communicating

When documenting discussions, be mindful of who might read the medical file. In public hospitals various people can access a patient file, so it is advisable to disclose only issues that are relevant and impact care but not give specifics. A good question to ask yourself is "Is this relevant to the nature of the work? What will it change?" For instance, if you are in a sexual health clinic and the patient has presented with sexual dysfunction, then details about the extent of dysfunction are clinically relevant for the medical file. On the other hand, in writing letters back to the referring physician, a high level of detail is unlikely to be relevant.

In facilitating communication with patients (and their partners) about sexual well-being, refer to the Further Reading section at the end of this chapter for useful patient resources.

Legal Responsibilities

It is important to be aware of your legal obligations. In some settings, clinicians are mandatory reporters—in other words, they can be prosecuted if they do not report crimes (e.g., underage sexual abuse) to the authorities. It is best to disclose your legal obligations with patients upfront. The usual consideration of psychotherapy boundaries also apply—for example, in most cases there will not be a need to physically touch the patient. It is good practice to gain consent to talk about private and personal issues.

Common Ethical Dilemmas

Things to consider in therapy include the competing needs of partners and/or their understanding of the impact of cancer and treatments. In the area of sexual dysfunction, this can be particularly important and is highlighted by the efficacy of couples-based interventions. In situations where patients are unpartnered, or in another situation where access to sexual activity may be hampered (e.g., disability), use of sex workers may be helpful—and giving the patient permission to explore new approaches can help to normalize this.

Policies

Sexual health and well-being is a basic human right. The World Health Organization asserts that human beings have "the rights to the highest attainable standard of health (including sexual health)" and have published "Sexual Health, Human Rights and the Law" to provide some general guidance (https://apps.who.int/iris/bitstream/handle/10665/175556/9789241564984_eng.pdf;jsessionid=7655253A81206BD1D68EDEC2B77664BA?sequence=1). The ASCO also has guidelines on interventions to address sexual problems in people with cancer (https://ascopubs.org/doi/full/10.1200/JCO.2017.75.8995). Ideally, a cancer center should have a sexual therapy clinic, or access to one, for management of problems with sexual adjustment in survivorship—however, this is not often the case.

Teams and Supervision

Supervision may focus on how to manage confronting conversations, working with couples, and managing conscientious objection (i.e., if you are not comfortable with something that the patients want to work on, then refer them to someone who is).

Training Modules

The e-learning interactive resource "Psychosexual Care of Women with Gynaecological Cancers" (PSGC) aims to provide health professionals with the knowledge, skills, and abilities to care for women who are at risk of, or are experiencing, psychosexual concerns and difficulties. The PSGC resource comprises a number of modules that present evidence-based information about sexuality, the psychosexual impact of cancer and its treatments, and the knowledge and skills required by health professionals to assess and manage psychosexual sequelae. Although developed in the gynecologic cancer setting, most of the modules will be relevant to health professionals working with any cancer population. It is available at https://education.eviq.org.au/courses/psychosexual-care-of-women-affected-by-gynaecologi.

"Starting the Conversation: Supporting Sexual Wellbeing for Women with Breast Cancer" has been developed to support health professionals initiate discussion about sexual well-being. It is available at https://canceraustralia.gov.au/sites/default/files/publications/2013_sexual_wellbeing_online_resource.pdf.

Principles of Sexual Rehabilitation for Individuals/Couples

- Incorporate routine and comprehensive clinical assessment for sexual changes and morbidity, particularly for groups with high-impact disease (e.g. breast, gynecologic, prostate, colorectal cancers).
- If desired by the patient, include partners in the sexual rehabilitation process.
- Consider "prehabilitation." Encourage the patient/couple to introduce sexual rehabilitation strategies before cancer treatment, before these become associated with sexual dysfunction.
- Intervene early (when medically safe). Although there is no consensus about specific timing of interventions, encourage the couple to recommence sexual activities and start interventions as early as possible.
- Multimodal integrated therapy is recommended. Since psychosexual issues are multifaceted, it is important to addresses the physical, emotional/psychological, and relationship elements of the sexual difficulty rather than relying on physical or biomedical interventions alone for the majority of patients/couples.
- Promote renegotiation and more flexible sexual practices and values, since sexual intimacy is always possible.
- Encourage sex despite low libido. Encourage the patient/couple to plan sexual encounters rather than waiting for the desire or urge to have sex.
- Foster realistic expectations regarding the extent and timeline for recovery of sexual function.

- Consider starting with the most effective treatment for sexual dysfunction (rather than the least invasive) to prevent demoralization and feelings of failure.
- Prepare patients to manage failures, and normalize the grieving process. For many patients return to baseline sexual function will not be possible.
- Establish sexual rehabilitation pathways and a referral network, with responsive services.[19,22]

References

1. Schover LR, van der Kaaij M, van Dorst E, et al. Sexual dysfunction and infertility as late effects of cancer treatment. *Eur J Cancer Suppl* 2014;12(1):41–53. doi:/10.1016/j.ejcsup.2014.03.004
2. Sears CS, Robinson JW, Walker LM. A comprehensive review of sexual health concerns after cancer treatment and the biopsychosocial treatment options available to female patients. *Eur J Cancer Care* 2018;27(2):e12738. doi:10.1111/ecc.12738
3. Boquiren VM, Esplen MJ, Wong J, et al. Sexual functioning in breast cancer survivors experiencing body image disturbance. *Psychooncology* 2016;25(1):66–76. doi:10.1002/pon.3819
4. Onujiogu N, Johnson T, Seo S, et al. Survivors of endometrial cancer: who is at risk for sexual dysfunction? *Gynecol Oncol* 2011;123(2):356–359. doi:10.1016/j.ygyno.2011.07.035
5. Lindau ST, Gavrilova N, Anderson D. Sexual morbidity in very long term survivors of vaginal and cervical cancer: a comparison to national norms. *Gynecol Oncol* 2007;106(2):413–418. doi:10.1016/j.ygyno.2007.05.017
6. Mitchell KR, Mercer CH, Ploubidis GB, et al. Sexual function in Britain: findings from the third National Survey of Sexual Attitudes and Lifestyles (Natsal-3). *Lancet* 2013;382(9907):1817–1829. doi:10.1016/S0140-6736(13)62366-1
7. Levin AO, Carpenter KM, Fowler JM, et al. Sexual morbidity associated with poorer psychological adjustment among gynecological cancer survivors. *Int J Gynecol Cancer* 2010;20(3):461–470. doi:10.1111/IGC.0b013e3181d24ce0
8. Burg MA, Adorno G, Lopez EDS, et al. Current unmet needs of cancer survivors: analysis of open-ended responses to the American Cancer Society Study of Cancer Survivors II. *Cancer* 2015;121(4):623–630. doi:10.1002/cncr.28951
9. Carter J, Lacchetti C, Andersen BL, et al. Interventions to address sexual problems in people with cancer: American Society of Clinical Oncology clinical practice guideline adaptation of Cancer Care Ontario guideline. *J Clin Oncol* 2018;36(5):492–511. doi:10.1200/jco.2017.75.8995
10. Basson R. A model of women's sexual arousal. *J Sex Marital Ther* 2002;28(1):1–10.
11. Hordern AJ, Street AF. Communicating about patient sexuality and intimacy after cancer: mismatched expectations and unmet needs. *Med J Austral* 2007;186(5):224–227.
12. Shaffer KM, Nelson CJ, DuHamel KN. Barriers to participation in a sexual health intervention for men following treatment for rectal and anal cancer. *Psychooncology* 2018;27(3):1082–1085.

13. Ussher JM, Perz J, Gilbert E, et al. Talking about sex after cancer: a discourse analytic study of health care professional accounts of sexual communication with patients. *Psychol Health* 2013;28(12):1370–1390.
14. Cherpak GL, Santos FC. Assessment of physicians' addressing sexuality in elderly patients with chronic pain. *Einstein (São Paulo)* 2016;14(2):178–184.
15. Wang K, Ariello K, Choi M, et al. Sexual healthcare for cancer patients receiving palliative care: a narrative review. *Ann Palliat Med* 2017;7(2):256–264.
16. Gilbert E, Perz J, Ussher JM. Talking about sex with health professionals: the experience of people with cancer and their partners. *Eur J Cancer Care* 2016;25(2):280–293. doi:10.1111/ecc.12216
17. White I. Managing the sexual consequences of cancer and its treatment. *CancerWorld* 2013;57:33–39.
18. Oberguggenberger AS, Nagele E, Inwald EC, et al. Phase 1–3 of the cross-cultural development of an EORTC questionnaire for the assessment of sexual health in cancer patients: the EORTC SHQ-22. *Cancer Med* 2018;7(3):635–645. doi:10.1002/cam4.1338
19. Walker LM, Wassersug RJ, Robinson JW. Psychosocial perspectives on sexual recovery after prostate cancer treatment. *Nature Rev Urol* 2015;12:167. doi:10.1038/nrurol.2015.29
20. Rowland DL. *Sexual Dysfunction in Men*. Göttingen, Germany: Hogrefe Publishing, 2012.
21. Rowland DL. *Sexual Dysfunction in Women*. Göttingen, Germany: Hogrefe Publishing, 2012.
22. Juraskova I. *Quality of Life/Quality of Sex: Psycho-sexual Adjustment Following Gynaecological Cancer*. Germany: VDM Verlag, 2009.
23. Bober SL, Varela VS. Sexuality in adult cancer survivors: challenges and intervention. *J Clin Oncol* 2012;30(30):3712–3719. doi:10.1200/jco.2012.41.7915
24. Frey AU, Sønksen J, Fode M. Neglected side effects after radical prostatectomy: a systematic review. *J Sex Med* 2014;11(2):374–385.
25. Yi JC, Syrjala KL. Sexuality after hematopoietic stem cell transplantation. *Cancer J* 2009;15(1):57–64. doi:10.1097/PPO.0b013e318198c758

Further Reading

Carter J, Lacchetti C, Andersen BL, et al. Clinical recommendations from an oncology perspective: interventions to address sexual problems in people with cancer: American Society of Clinical Oncology's clinical practice guideline adaptation of Cancer Care Ontario guideline. *J Clin Oncol* 2018;36(5):492–511. doi:10.1200/JCO.2017.75.8995

Useful Patient Resources

The Cancer Council Australia has some useful general patient information about sexuality, intimacy, and cancer, in particular a pamphlet that describes the impact and the treatments in detail. It includes diagrams that can be used when referring to male and female anatomy, information about communicating with partners, and a question checklist to help patients start conversations with health professionals: https://www.cancercouncil.com.au/cancer-information/managing-cancer-side-effects/sexuality-intimacy/

Books/Resources That May Be Helpful to Women

- *Woman Cancer Sex* by Anne Katz: Specifically written for women with cancer; covers sexual functioning, depression, physical and emotional feelings, and specific strategies to treat the problems.
- *Sexy After Cancer: Meeting Your Inner Aphrodite on the Breast Cancer Journey* by Barbara Musser: The author discusses sex after breast cancer. Note that the author's blog URL mentioned in this book, sexyaftercancer.com, redirects to a commercial site selling bras designed for women with breast cancer.
- *Sex for One: The Joy of Self-Loving* by Betty Dodson: This guidebook takes the shame out of self-love.
- *Where Did My Libido Go?* by Rosie King: Written for women who feel little or no desire for sex.
- An Australian app provides access to reliable up-to-date information (videos, webinars, leaflets, podcasts, etc.) on topics that are relevant to women (including sexuality and intimacy) with breast or gynecologic cancers: https://counterpart.org.au/information/navigators/

Books/Resources That May Be Helpful to Men

- *Man Cancer Sex* by Anne Katz: Explores how men are affected by a diagnosis of cancer and how they can seek help
- *Facing the Tiger: A Guide for Men with Prostate Cancer and the People Who Love Them* by Suzanne Chambers: Provides practical strategies to help cope with the emotional and psychological stress of living with prostate cancer, including sexual dysfunction.
- *Too Fast? Learn to Last Longer* by Michael Lowy and Brett McCann: Provides useful self-help information about ejaculation disorders, particularly premature ejaculation.
- LIVEStrong website: https://www.livestrong.org/we-can-help/finishing-treatment/male-sexual-health-after-cancer
- TrueNth is a US-based Movember initiative that helps men navigate their prostate cancer journey and includes some sexual health information: https://us.truenth.org/

Books/Resources That May Be Helpful to Couples

- *Resurrecting Sex: Solving Sexual Problems and Revolutionizing Your Relationship* by David Schnarch: A book about how couples can work on their sexual relationship.
- *Good Loving, Great Sex: Finding Balance When Your Sex Drives Differ* by Rosie King: Provides readers with the skills to build a sensual and satisfying sexual relationship, despite differing sex drives.
- *The Sex Diaries: Why Women Go Off Sex and Other Bedroom Battles* by Bettina Arndt: Proposes a new approach of how couples can enjoy regular sex and sustain loving relationships, based on diaries of 98 couples.

Chapter 6

Psychological Treatment of Individual Sexual Dysfunction

Daniela Wittmann

Learning Objectives

After reading this chapter the clinician will be able to:

1. Recognize the typical sexual side effects of cancer treatment
2. Understand and empathize with the emotional responses experienced by individuals with cancer and their partners that typically accompany sexual dysfunctions and how those might affect the relationship
3. Be able to formulate a biopsychosocial diagnosis
4. Guide the patient through shared clinical decision-making and options for clinical management
5. Prescribe appropriately three interventions that will enable an individual with cancer to optimally manage a sexual relationship

Background Evidence

Sexual problems after cancer treatment are highly prevalent in both men and women. Studies have measured sexual symptoms at various time points after treatment in long-term survivorship: Approximately 40% of adolescent and young adult cancer survivors, over 78% of survivors treated with prostate surgery, and over 60% of survivors treated with radiation for localized prostate cancer report sexual problems 2 years after treatment,[1,2] 65% of men and 74% of women with colorectal cancer report sexual dysfunction 6 months after treatment,[3] and 60% of women with breast cancer experience sexual problems over 10 years after treatment.[4]

The literature on sexual problems in cancer is somewhat uneven. While most research has been done on cancers that can be clearly linked to sexual problems, such as breast, colorectal, or prostate cancer, it is important to recognize that treatments for other cancers, not intuitively associated with sexual dysfunction, can be just as challenging for sexual intimacy. For example, treatment for head and neck cancer can leave the patient without saliva that is needed for kissing, and odors emanating from the mouth after treatment may make mouth-to-mouth contact unpleasant.[5] More evidence documenting sexual dysfunctions in different cancers is needed.

Sexual problems most frequently reported by men with cancer are changes in libido or sexual interest, erectile and orgasmic function, and penile shrinkage. Women most frequently report low or no sexual interest, vaginal dryness, and pain with intercourse. Gay and bisexual men report inability to assume their usual roles in anal sex either because of erections insufficiently hard for penetration or because changes in the tissues of the anus prevent a comfortable or sensitive receptive anal sex experience.

The concept of sexual dysfunction, most often used in the literature to designate sexual problems, has been evolving with initial emphasis, in the second half of the 20th century, on physiologic dysfunction and sexual satisfaction. Vroege et al. described sexual dysfunction as "the various ways in which an individual is unable to participate in a sexual relationship as he or she would wish," including lack or loss of sexual desire, sexual aversion disorder, failure of genital response (erectile dysfunction, rapid or dry ejaculation, poor vaginal lubrication), orgasmic dysfunction, nonorganic vaginismus, nonorganic dyspareunia, and excessive sexual drive.[6] In addition, original perspectives on sexual dysfunctions differentiated between physiologic and psychological causation. A consensus statement from the Fourth International Consultation on Sexual Medicine in 2015 recognized that attempts to dichotomize sexual problems into body and mind dualism were not effective and emphasized that the etiology of sexual problems is not fully understood: "Sexual dysfunction concepts are largely descriptive and aspects of the physiologic sexual experience are clearly influenced by psychosocial factors" and vice versa.[7]

Today we understand that sexuality has physiologic, psychological, social, as well as cultural components, as described by Bober and Varela.[8] Men and women respond with feelings of distress, a sense of loss and grief, depression, anxiety, embarrassment, and loss of sexual confidence as they attempt to come to terms with cancer treatment–related altered sexual function, body image, and sense of sexual self. For many, return to baseline sexual function with which they are familiar is no longer possible. Developing a new method for obtaining sexual pleasure and sharing it in a relationship becomes a focus and a challenge in long-term survivorship.[9,10]

Expanding the lens to include partners is important in the assessment and treatment of sexual issues in cancer. Partners report feelings of distress as they become caregivers for cancer patients who have experienced a loss of sexual function and sexual confidence after cancer treatment.[11,12] They report grief about the patient's sexual losses and the implications of those losses for them. In order to protect and retain their sex lives, cancer patients and their partners must engage in problem solving that includes sexual communication, use of sexual aids, and some degree of experimentation with new sexual activities. The goal of such problem solving is to build competence and reassurance that sex can be again pleasurable and unselfconscious. For many couples, sexual communication may need to be a newly learned skill that they may not have needed or used in the past.[13] Single men and women have unique challenges that are outlined in Box 6.1.

> **Box 6.1 Special Considerations for Single Men and Women**
>
> - Single men and women worry about entering a new relationship given their cancer history and need for assisted sexual function.
> - To avoid unnecessary rejection, single men and women need to learn to assess a potential new partner's receptivity to their situation.
> - Single men and women have to develop confidence that they can satisfy a partner sexually despite their own altered sexual function.

Finally, given that cancer and its care affects men and women with different sexual orientations (see Chapter 3) and religious and ethnic backgrounds, it is necessary to be mindful about what is an acceptable topic in discussions about sexual concerns, who should best have those conversations, and what solutions fit best with a particular patient's sexual practice (heterosexual, gay, bisexual) and religious or ethnic frame of reference.[14]

Presenting Problems

Key Symptoms and Signs

Cancer treatments push patients' sexuality into an experience associated with aging. It is common for patients to frame sexual losses in this way with all the implications of having to come to terms with life-altering functional decline. Although sexual symptoms are similar regardless of cancer and treatment type, it is useful to have a sense of the typical symptoms associated with a particular cancer and its treatment (Table 6.1).

Sexual side effects of cancer treatment are a topic that is important to discuss with patients and their partners prior to treatment so that the patient can know what to expect. While it may seem that, in the context of the threat of cancer, bringing up the topic of sexuality would be of low priority to patients, this is generally not true. In some cases, such as in prostate cancer, understanding the sexual side effects can influence the type of treatment a patient will choose. In all cases, it is helpful to the patient and to the healthcare provider to understand, during pretreatment discussions, whether sexuality is important to the patient and partner. Regardless of the frequency of sexual activity alone or with a partner, or whether the patient's sexual activity includes penetration, some men and women value their sexuality and want to protect it from the effects of their cancer treatment to the degree that it is possible. In some cases, this can lead to including, in planning cancer surgeries, efforts to spare nerves that govern men's erections, and organs, such as vaginas and ovaries that allow women to avoid the transition into menopause as a consequence of treatment. The goal of cancer eradication always trumps these plans, but surgeons increasingly recognize the importance of patients' quality of life after cancer treatment. Similar considerations can be included in discussions of treatment with pelvic radiation. In addition, a sexual

Table 6.1 Typical Sexual Problems by Cancer Type

Cancer Type	Physiologic	Psychological	Relationship	Sexual Orientation Consideration	Religion/Ethnicity Consideration
Breast	Loss of breast; hormonal therapy: diminished sexual interest, vaginal dryness, dyspareunia, changes in sexual sensitivity, orgasmic difficulty	Feelings of loss, grief, diminished sexual confidence, distress about body image, guilt about diminished sexual interest, decision-making about breast, reconstruction, fear of abandonment by partner	Poor communication, lack of problem solving and help seeking, partner distress, avoidance of sexual activity	Ambivalence about breast reconstruction	Cultural meaning of mastectomy and breast reconstruction
Colorectal—men	Erectile dysfunction, possible fecal incontinence	Feelings of loss, grief, diminished sexual confidence, distress about body image and masculinity, shame and embarrassment about fecal incontinence	Poor communication, anxiety/disgust about fecal incontinence, lack of problem solving and help seeking, partner distress, avoidance of sexual activity	Concerns about firm erection and integrity of anal tissues relevant to anal sex	Cultural meaning of erectile dysfunction, options for treatments and for fecal incontinence
Colorectal—women	Diminished sexual interest, vaginal dryness, dyspareunia, changes in sexual sensitivity, orgasmic difficulty, vaginal stenosis if radiation treatment was given	Feelings of loss, grief, diminished sexual confidence, distress about body image, guilt about diminished sexual interest	Poor communication, anxiety/disgust about fecal incontinence, lack of problem solving and help seeking, partner distress, avoidance of sexual activity	None	Cultural meaning of fecal incontinence

Bladder—men (if invasive, involves removal of bladder and prostate)	Erectile dysfunction, orgasmic dysfunction, fatigue-related low interest, urinary incontinence	Feelings of loss, grief, diminished sexual confidence, distress about body image and masculinity, shame and embarrassment about urinary incontinence	Poor communication, anxiety about urinary incontinence, lack of problem solving and help seeking, partner distress, avoidance of sexual activity	Concerns about firm erection and integrity of anal tissues relevant to anal sex	Cultural meaning of erectile dysfunction, options for treatment, urinary diversions
Bladder—women (if invasive, involves removal of bladder, possibly uterus and ovaries, vagina)	Diminished sexual interest, vaginal dryness, dyspareunia, changes in sexual sensitivity, orgasmic difficulty, vaginal stenosis if radiation treatment was given	Feelings of loss, grief, diminished confidence, distress about body image, guilt about diminished interest	Poor communication, anxiety about urinary incontinence, lack of problem solving and help seeking, partner distress, avoidance of sexual activity	None	Cultural meaning of urinary diversions
Head and neck	Difficulty kissing due to dry mouth, thickened saliva, mouth sores, loss of teeth/jaw bone, lymphedema of the neck, fatigue, diminished sexual interest	Feelings of loss, grief, diminished sexual confidence, distress about body image, guilt about diminished sexual interest and inability to kiss, feelings about human papillomavirus (HPV) transmission as a result of sexual contact/potential infidelity	Poor communication, lack of problem solving and help seeking, partner distress and concerns about potential infidelity, avoidance of sexual activity	Inability to perform oral sex	Cultural meaning of visible physical changes due to cancer and potential infidelity

Table 6.1 Continued

Cancer Type	Physiologic	Psychological	Relationship	Sexual Orientation Consideration	Religion/Ethnicity Consideration
Prostate, localized	Erectile dysfunction, orgasmic dysfunction, urinary incontinence or irritability, penile shrinkage and potential for the development of Peyronie disease if treated with surgery, bowel dysfunction if treated with radiation	Feelings of loss, grief, diminished sexual confidence, distress about body image and masculinity, shame and embarrassment about urinary and bowel problems	Poor communication, lack of problem solving and help seeking, partner distress, avoidance of sexual activity	Concerns about firm erection and integrity of anal tissues relevant to anal sex, significance of the loss of ejaculation for erotic expression, stigma about sexual dysfunction in the gay community	Cultural meaning of erectile dysfunction, options for treatment, urinary diversions
Prostate, advanced	Diminished sexual interest, erectile dysfunction, genital shrinkage, orgasmic dysfunction, breast growth, body hair loss, feminizing redistribution of body fat	Feelings of loss, grief, diminished sexual confidence, distress about body image and masculinity, shame and embarrassment about altered sexual self	Poor communication, lack of problem solving and help seeking, partner distress, great potential for loss of sexual activity	Loss of sexual viability, particularly for single men	Cultural meaning of sexual changes

Testicular	Loss of testicle, potential erectile dysfunction, retrograde ejaculation	Feelings of loss, grief, diminished sexual confidence, distress about body image and masculinity	Poor communication, lack of problem solving and help seeking, partner distress, avoidance of sexual activity	Concerns about loss of ejaculation	Cultural meaning of loss of fertility
Uterine and ovarian	Loss of uterus and ovaries; diminished sexual interest, vaginal dryness, dyspareunia, changes in sexual sensitivity, orgasmic difficulty	Feelings of loss, grief, diminished sexual confidence, distress about body image, guilt about diminished sexual interest	Poor communication, lack of problem solving and help seeking, partner distress, avoidance of sexual activity	None	Cultural meaning of loss of fertility
Cervical	Loss of cervix, sometimes loss of ovaries and shortening of the vagina; diminished sexual interest, vaginal dryness, dyspareunia, changes in sexual sensitivity, orgasmic difficulty	Feelings of loss, grief, diminished sexual confidence, distress about body image, guilt about diminished sexual interest	Poor communication, lack of problem solving and help seeking, partner distress, avoidance of sexual activity	None	Cultural meaning of loss of fertility

health assessment prior to treatment and afterwards can direct the kind of support that the patient will require.

The mechanisms through which sexual dysfunction might develop vary by treatment. *Surgery* in the pelvis for prostate, bladder, and colorectal cancer damages nerves responsible for erectile function in men. The removal of the prostate in prostate and bladder cancer leads to the loss of ejaculatory fluid. Surgery for bladder, colorectal, and gynecologic cancers in women can lead to premature menopause, diminishing sexual interest, and pain with intercourse due to loss of vaginal lubrication, particularly if ovaries are removed. Extensive surgery can result in difficulty with intercourse if the vaginal vault has been shortened. *Radiation* to the pelvis can lead to erectile dysfunction in men and vaginal stenosis and loss of lubrication in women. If *hormonal deprivation* is a part of cancer treatment, as, for example, in prostate and breast cancer, sexual interest decreases and orgasms can become weaker. Other symptoms, such as fatigue and irritability, add obstacles to sexual activity and pleasure. Most men develop genital shrinkage, and women's vaginal lubrication is further diminished. Urinary leakage and bowel leakage, which are present after some pelvic cancer treatments, interfere with the experience of pleasure and need to be managed during sexual activity. Finally, systemic *chemotherapy* can lead to similar functional difficulties, and, at least temporarily, fatigue affects interest in sexual activity.

A comprehensive evaluation will include an assessment of the patient's understanding of the treatment's sexual side effects, the patient's level of distress about functional changes, the status of the patient's grief response, and the patient's concerns about the ability to function in a sexual relationship with confidence despite functional losses. It will be necessary to evaluate whether the patient's expectations of functional recovery are realistic, as overly optimistic expectations will lead to anxiety and depression—emotional states that interfere with sexual recovery. Including the partner, if available, is essential as the partner must have similar understanding of the sexual side effects of treatment, realistic expectations of the patient's sexual recovery, and an opportunity to discuss his or her sexual concerns in the context of the cancer treatment. Including the partner will make apparent the ease of or barriers to communication about sexual concerns within the couple in general and in the cancer context in particular. Studies have shown that patients and partners who protect each other from cancer-related difficult topics tend to evidence poorer couple functioning. If possible, the partner's sexual function should be assessed as well so as to have a baseline understanding of preexisting sexual issues and the couple's coping success or lack thereof. Sexual orientation and sociocultural factors must be addressed in the evaluation so that patients can feel confident that their needs will be understood and addressed.

The level and complexity of the patient's support needs will depend on the extent of the sexual changes after treatment. While low or no libido may be distressing, it is generally the genital symptoms that cause the greatest sense of loss because they directly affect the patient's ability to feel sexual pleasure. Loss of body parts such as testes and breasts is also influential, although they may be thought of as affecting more significantly a person's body image and feelings of attractiveness and masculinity or femininity rather than his or her sexuality.

Clinicians should be alert to confounding issues that can lead to misdiagnosis and inappropriate treatment:

- Low testosterone levels in men can present as low libido, erectile dysfunction, fatigue, even depression. Patients and clinicians may interpret these symptoms from a psychological perspective. A test of bioavailable testosterone can help clarify the origin of the symptoms. In most cases, testosterone can be supplemented, even in some men with nonaggressive, localized prostate cancer. Similarly, low estrogen levels in women, already present in postmenopausal women, can have a role in reports of low libido, fatigue, vaginal dryness, and pain with intercourse. In women whose cancer is not hormonally driven, hormone replacement therapy can be considered. Patients should be advised to discuss the possibility of hormonal supplementation with their oncologists and, if deemed appropriate, seek referral to either andrologists (men) or gynecologists (women) for specialty care.
- Treatment for depression or anxiety with selective serotonin reuptake inhibitors (SSRIs) can present as anorgasmia (difficulty reaching orgasm). Understanding the biology of these medications' interference with the sexual response cycle can lead to a productive discussion about how to manage depression/anxiety and sexual issues optimally. Antidepressants with no sexual side effects (e.g., bupropion hydrochloride or mirtazapine) can be considered.
- Carefully sorting out the contribution of biologic, psychological, and relationship issues to sexual dysfunction is necessary before optimal treatment can be recommended.

Case Study

Mr. C, a 65-year-old African American married man, was a prostate cancer survivor of 4 years. He developed erectile dysfunction after cancer treatment and wanted to try erectile aids postoperatively. Increasingly invasive erectile aids were prescribed by his urologist. Phosphodiesterase type 5 inhibitors did not work at all, which was not unusual in this situation. Mr. C tried transurethral suppositories with prostaglandin E, then intracavernosal injections. Each of these methods was initially successful for about 2 months but then failed. Given this result, Mr. C requested, and was provided with, a penile implant. He returned after 3 months. According to him, the implant, which had worked well initially, began failing. Mr. C was not able to explain why, reporting only that it was not working. A physical examination did not reveal a mechanical problem with the implant itself. Since the couple's sexual repertoire was limited to intercourse, Mr. C felt particularly despondent. He was referred for a psychosexual evaluation, which revealed that Mr. C had a very unhappy marriage. His wife had rejected him sexually for many years and chose other lovers. Since his prostate cancer treatment, she was unwilling to undertake any alternative sexual activity and was generally not interested in participating in his sexual recovery. In trying various erectile aids, he hoped to overcome his wife's disinterest. When he was unable to do so, he became discouraged and wished to try a new erectile aid. At the time of the psychosexual evaluation, Mr. C was discouraged, expressing feelings of frustration and hopelessness. He said that he was afraid that his wife would leave him. The evaluation helped Mr. C recognize that the issue was not a matter of finding the right erectile aid but coming to terms with his marital history, acknowledging lifelong sexual losses. He was offered individual sex therapy to work through grief and mourning about his marriage with the goal of becoming more confident and able to make decisions about his future as a man and sexual partner in the context of his cancer-related sexual health status. He accepted the recommendation. Individual treatment resulted in his grieving for the long-term relationship and sexual losses, developing confidence, leaving his wife, and starting a new relationship that provided him with more mutuality and sexual compatibility.

Investigations for Key Differential Diagnosis

Key Differentials

- *Discussion of the typical sexual side effects of a particular cancer and its treatment* is a necessary starting point because it establishes an objective baseline for the patient who may misconstrue those side effects as psychological responses.
- *Sexual function assessment* will delineate the problems that the individual is experiencing physiologically. Using validated measures and starting before treatment can be helpful both as a record of the change and as a method for starting the discussion of anticipated sexual side effects of cancer treatment. General sexual function assessments that have been used in clinical practice are the International Index of Erectile Function[15] and the Female Sexual Function Index.[16] Disease-specific measures with sexual function domains are also available, for example the Expanded Prostate Cancer Index Composite (EPIC)[17] or the Bladder Cancer Index (BCI).[18] The Reported Outcome Measures Information System (PROMIS)[19] has a sexual health manual with items that evaluate not only sexual function but also sexual activity, use of sexual aids, sexual interest, and satisfaction with sex life. All can provide valuable information about the patient's functional status.
- *Pain with penetration assessment* for women may include a physical therapy assessment to identify scaring, vaginal atrophy, vaginal stenosis, pelvic floor dysfunction, and other muscular issues. Pelvic floor assessment may be useful for men if they have pain with orgasm or erectile dysfunction. Assessment for men may include an anal exam to identify muscles compromised by radiation therapy.
- *Assessment of distress, the grief process, and potential depression and anxiety* in reaction to sexual losses helps not only with the assessment of the psychological state, but also with the possible additional influences on sexual

function. The assessment can include the use of validated measures, such as the Patient Health Questionnaire-9[20] for depression.
- *Assessment of the patient's sexual history and current relationship* through discussion with the individual patient or with the couple elucidates contributing historical, partner, and relationship factors that would have to be addressed in a psychosexual intervention. This includes the partner's response to the patient's sexual changes, partner sexual function, couple sexual history, sexual communication, and sexual repertoire.

Additional Assessments

- *Comorbidities assessment* is necessary to account for additional negative effects of conditions such as diabetes or Parkinson disease on sexual function and sexual experience.
- *Medical treatments* for comorbid conditions, such as SSRIs, beta blockers, and dopamine enhancers, have been shown to be implicated in sexual problems.
- *History of mental illness and sexual abuse* helps determine potential factors in poor coping.
- *Substance use assessment* is necessary as substances such as alcohol, amphetamines, barbiturates, marijuana, nicotine, and opiates diminish sexual function and the experience of sexual pleasure.

Setting realistic expectations, based on the assessment, is a key component of the initial assessment (Box 6.2).

Distinguishing between depression and grief is important because many people label sad and discouraged feelings as depression. Reactions to the changes in sexual function and sexual relationships can be intense. Patients can be confused about what they are experiencing. The major difference between depression and grief is most easily identified as the availability of active energy. A depressed person finds it difficult to get out of bed in the morning and generally finds himself or herself not experiencing any interest or pleasure in people or activities. In

---

Box 6.2 Setting Realistic Expectations

- Setting realistic expectations is a part of assessment
- To the degree that it can be anticipated, it is important to provide the patient with information about the severity of the impact of the cancer and its treatment on sexual function and likelihood of sexual function recovery.
- For example, hormonal treatment and some pelvic cancer treatments result in irreversible changes in sexual function.
- Promoting realistic expectations of outcomes sets the stage for the likely need to use sexual aids.

contrast, while grief is profoundly painful and can include feelings of hopelessness, there is usually still an ability to enjoy relationships and activities. The intense feelings of grief come and go in waves. Patients find the distinction helpful, even energizing, particularly if grief is normalized.

Suicidal feelings can arise as an aspect of both deep depression and intense grief. Feelings such as not being "good enough" as a lover with sexual dysfunction, fears of rejection or abandonment that lower self-worth, and hopelessness or concern that there will never be another sexually active relationship could induce such suicidal thoughts. Clinicians must recognize and assess potential for suicidal thoughts and plans and follow procedures for appropriate management).[21]

Guilt in response to altered sexual function because of perceived inability to be a good sexual partner must be considered. Patients may withdraw and avoid sexual interactions for fear of being unattractive, less feminine or masculine, or unable to satisfy their partner. This response must be teased out beyond the feelings of loss because it is one that can be addressed in psychosexual treatment.

Biopsychosocial Formulation

A comprehensive assessment takes into account the physiologic, psychological, and relationship aspects of the patient's presentation to make decisions about appropriate treatment (see Box 6.3).

Box 6.3 A Biopsychosocial Formulation

A biopsychosocial formulation includes the following:
- Pre-existing physiologic sexual dysfunction such as low libido or erectile or orgasmic dysfunction for men or postmenopausal low libido and vaginal dryness or orgasmic dysfunction in older women or similar symptoms in younger women, not related to menopause
- Cancer treatment–related sexual side effects, including the patient's understanding of their short-term or long-term persistence
- The impact of comorbidities and their medical treatments on sexual function
- Patient's current coping (identify strengths and vulnerabilities)
- Mental health or substance use issues that might affect coping
- The impact of the sexual side effects on the partner and the relationship and any preexisting relationship problems
- The impact of sexual orientation and cultural issues and potential stigma and discrimination on clinical management.

Clinical Management

Clinical management of sexual problems can be complex as one must consider at once the physiologic, psychological, and relationship aspects of sexuality. This also means that the best approach to management is multidisciplinary. Which disciplines will be needed for any given patient will depend on the assessment of the problems. Members of the following disciplines may be needed: a relevant cancer specialist, a sexual health expert, a mental health expert, a nurse who is trained in sexual health care, a physical therapist who specializes in the area of the patient's body that needs attention (e.g., in pelvic floor rehabilitation), a sexual medicine urologist, a gynecologist, and a primary care physician. Collaboration between members of these disciplines will be critical to the success of the patient's psychosexual recovery during and after cancer treatment. Figure 6.1 depicts key assessments and decision points for clinical management.

Psychosocial Interventions

Managing expectations of what is possible as patients work on sexual recovery is a vital aspect of the process and must be addressed repeatedly. Patients want to know not only what they can expect, but also where they stand in relation to others. In a sense, they wish to know that their sexual problems are normal, given their cancer and its treatment. The feeling of "not being alone" can enhance motivation and ultimately confidence. This may be done individually, with the partner present, or in a group setting. If possible, the discussion of expectations is best done prior to treatment because this can reduce feelings of loss and facilitate the grief process (Table 6.2).

Supportive Counseling

Supportive counseling can be beneficial for the majority of patients, as many have strengths they can use in their recovery. This includes listening to their concerns, accepting their feelings of loss and frustration, and not expecting them to quickly transition into accepting that their lives have been unalterably changed. Inviting partners to participate in some sessions gives both members of the couple an opportunity to express their feelings about the changes and to use humor, practicality, and their strengths as individuals and as a couple in their work toward managing their sexual lives in a new way. Individual counseling and group counseling have both been shown to lead to more successful incorporation of sexual aids. This is particularly true if the partner is incorporated in the counseling.

Both the patient and the partner will need support in accepting sexual aids because the sexual life of both has changed. Generally speaking, patients will be interested in learning how they might enhance their sexual function. For men, that often means medical and mechanical erectile aids; for women, this means vaginal lubricants, vibrators, and dilators. However, research has shown that many patients do not use or do not persist in using sexual aids. This is largely due to the fact that in using them, patients grieve the loss of spontaneous sex, have to overcome negative feelings about the use of sexual aids, and, in some cases, such as when men use erectile aids and women use vaginal dilators, experience pain or discomfort before they see positive results.

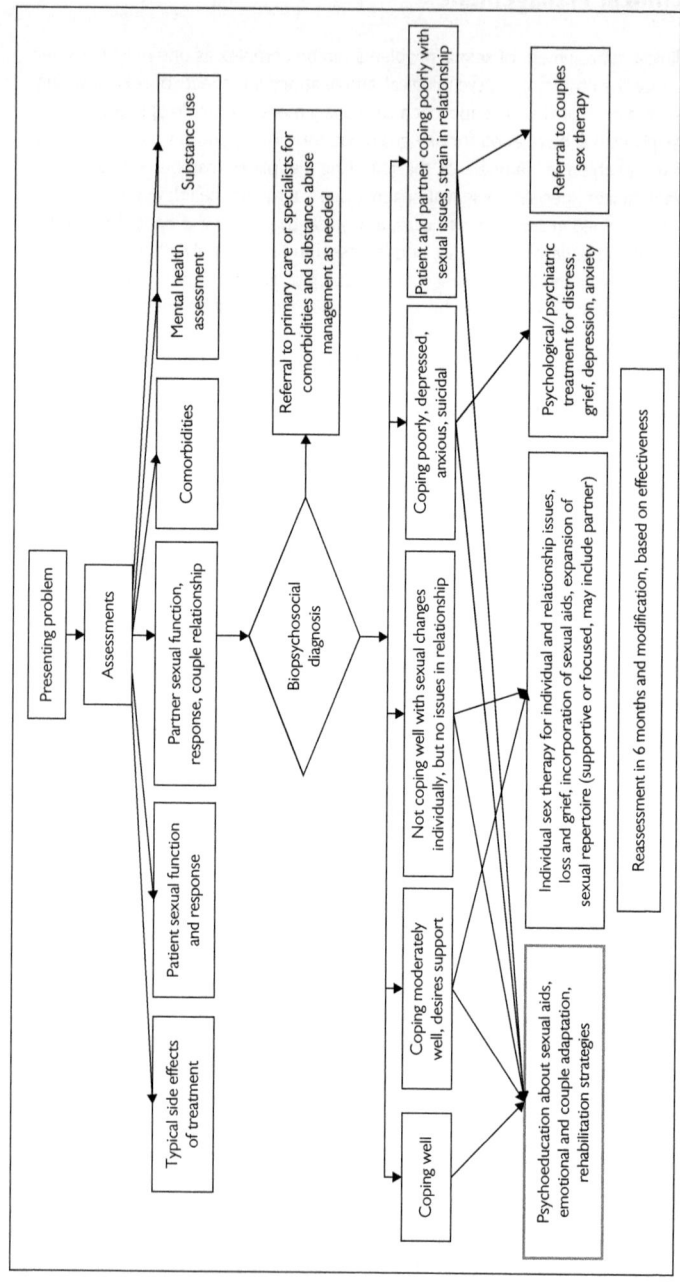

Figure 6.1 Flow-chart of assessment and formulation to determine optimal intervention plans

Table 6.2 Psychosocial Interventions

Intervention	Format	Frequency	Desired Outcome
Psychoeducation to learn about sexual side effects, rehabilitation, emotional and relationship impacts, manage expectations	Individual patient, patient and partner, or group setting for patients and partners	With individual patients, during each appointment before and after treatment	Realistic expectations of sexual function recovery
Supportive counseling to witness grief about sexual losses, expand sexual repertoire, empower single patients to begin a new relationship; relies on individual and relationship strengths	Patient, may invite partner	Tailored individually; starts monthly, then decreasing frequency	Acceptance of sexual aids as needed, engagement or reengagement in sexual relationship
Individual sex therapy to address deep grief, loss of confidence, barriers to sexual recovery	Patient	Weekly, at least initially	Acceptance of sexual losses, use of sexual aids if needed, increased sexual confidence
Mindfulness meditation to increase sexual arousal	Individual patient or group setting	Weekly, time limited	Ability to focus on sexual arousal without intrusive negative thoughts interfering
Sensate focus exercise to reengage comfortably in sensual and sexual activity	Preferably as a couple, but can be used as self-exploration	Tailored individually	Discovery of sensual and sexual body foci, ability to overcome embarrassment and anxiety and focus on pleasure
Expansion of sexual repertoire	Individual patient, may invite partner	Tailored individually; starts monthly, then decreasing frequency	Increasing sources of sexual pleasure for the individual and in the relationship
Couples sex therapy	Patient and partner	Referral	Resolution of long-term issues, improved communication and sexual relationship

In patients with some cancers, supportive counseling includes discussing interfering factors, such as urinary or fecal incontinence. This is particularly mortifying for patients who feel ashamed and fearful of inflicting their challenges on the partner. Both the patient and the partner can learn to manage these side effects together as they grow to accept them as either a temporary or permanent aspect of their sexual intimacy. Patients can be taught strategies for emptying the bladder or bowels, or disguising stomas prior to sexual activity can help. Experience has shown that patients can cope with these side effects if they can come to terms with them and both members of the couple can adopt a practical approach to management.

In supportive counseling, single patients can practice bringing up their cancer to a new potential partner and assessing his or her ability to accept a relationship with a cancer survivor. If reassured, they can practice discussing their altered sexual function. It is critical that patients initiate these conversations when they feel reasonably confident that they can be good lovers and satisfy their partners. Finally, they can practice sexual communication in which they ask for what they need sexually, now that sex is not spontaneous and requires new competencies.

Individual Sex Therapy

Individual sex therapy can be helpful in addressing patients' intense, persistent feelings about the loss of sexual function, changes in body image, and loss of sexual confidence. Issues from the patient's earlier life, such as sexual abuse or personal feelings of failure, may need to be explored before the current sexual issues can be successfully addressed. Witnessing grief, normalizing the experience, and working through past issues that act as barriers can reduce anxiety and enhance willingness to explore new strategies for managing a sexual experience and relationship successfully and competently despite functional deficits after cancer treatment. This is especially valuable for single patients who anticipate dating and finding a new partner with trepidation. As in supportive counseling, patients can practice having conversations with potential partners in a way that projects confidence about their abilities as sexual partners and minimizes the likelihood of rejection.

Mindfulness Meditation

Mindfulness meditation has been shown to enhance focus on arousal in women, reduce stress, and improve sexual satisfaction. The goal is not to allow negative intrusive thoughts to interfere with sexual arousal. While it has been mostly implemented with women who do not have cancer, cancer survivors have also shown benefit. Mindfulness meditation can be used during all phases of illness. Success using both group and individual approaches has been reported. Treatment typically has a time-limited format of several weeks. Patients can be encouraged to use mindfulness to reduce anxiety as they approach sexual encounters.

Sensate Focus Exercises

Sensate focus exercises are recommended for couples who are tentative about resuming sexual activity after cancer treatment. Generally best guided by a sex therapist familiar with the relevant cancer issues, these exercises begin with nonsexual, sensual touch of areas mutually agreed on by the couple; sexual activity is not pursued at first. These exercises include a discussion of the feelings generated by touching and being touched. As comfort with touching increases, the exercises can progress to sexual and genital touching, and eventually to penetrative sex. This approach can be also used with an individual patient who is exploring his or her sensual and sexual sensitivity that was altered by cancer treatment. Patients who have a partner for whom this approach is appropriate may accept a referral to a sex therapist. Some patients who are comfortable in their relationships may try to practice sensate focus at home on their own but will likely benefit the most if this is done in sex therapy.

Expanded Sexual Repertoire

Expansion of sexual repertoire means not only using new strategies to enhance sexual pleasure but also returning to strategies practiced earlier in the relationship. For example, in their usual sexual activity, long-term couples may quickly move to intercourse without much foreplay. When sexual function is more fragile and there is a need for more stimulation, returning to caressing, manual stimulation, and oral sex can be helpful to enhance arousal and sexual pleasure. These may be new strategies for those who have been intercourse-dependent throughout their relationship. The use of vibrators promotes blood flow and enhances sexual sensitivity for both men and women. Although this is not a strategy generally seen in heterosexual couples, some gay couples have reported that they found incorporating a new lover into their sexual activity was a way to maintain optimal sexual pleasure for all parties. Sensitivity to cultural and religious preferences is critical here, but most individuals appreciate suggestions for improving their experience and the experience of their partner.

Couples Sex Therapy

Couples sex therapy can be very beneficial to cancer patients as it immediately addresses a barrier to sexual recovery: communication about sexual problems and sexual rehabilitation. It recognizes the partner as an important stakeholder in the management of sexual issues, which in turn supports the legitimacy of the patient's sexual concerns. Couples sex therapy is often recommended for patients when the sexual health assessment suggests that there are additional or preexisting couple problems that are likely to impede sexual recovery. Couples sex therapy uses a number of strategies: grief work to recognize sexual losses, cognitive-behavioral strategies to overcome resistance to the use of sexual aids, encouragement of sexual communication to facilitate mutuality, and experimentation to expand sexual repertoire. In couples sex therapy, patients and partners are encouraged to reserve time at home to focus on their sexual relationship and to experiment with new behaviors to "re-eroticize" sexual interactions and foster mutuality.

Biomedical Interventions

Sexual aids for men include phosphodiesterase type 5 inhibitors, vacuum erectile devices, intracavernosal injections, intraurethral suppositories, and penile prostheses. Men should be made aware of all the aids and should be encouraged to try them until they find the most satisfactory approach (Table 6.3).

Sexual aids for women include the use of vaginal lubricants, moisturizers, and dilators to increase comfort with penetration. Topical, local hormonal replacement, obtained by prescription, can also make a contribution for women whose cancers are not hormone-responsive. Vibrators and clitoral pumps improve orgasmic function by increasing blood flow. Flibanserin, a

Table 6.3 Guide to Sexual Aids for Patients

Men—Erectile Function Aids

Treatment	Dose	Side Effects	Contraindications
Vacuum erection device	NA	Bruising if over-pump (petechiae)	Peyronie curvature, sickle cell anemia
Phosphodiesterase type 5 inhibitors (prescription by a urologist or primary care physician)	Sildenafil, avanafil, vardenafil: once daily either 50 mg or 100 mg. Tadalafil: daily 5 mg, 20 mg per 36 hours	Headache, facial flushing, nasal congestion, upset stomach	Concomitant nitrates or alpha blockers. Cardiology consult for history of arrhythmias, stroke, heart attack. Hematology Consult for history of priapism
Intracavernosal injections (prescription by a urologist, must be taught in the urologist's office)	Prostaglandin E or papaverin. Dosing in micrograms, individually determined	Temporary penile and/or testicular pain after orgasm, headache, flu symptoms, Peyronie curvature can develop	Requires manual dexterity to administer injections. Caution with anticoagulant use. Caution with history of priapism. Cardiology consult for history of arrhythmias, stroke, heart attack
Intraurethral tablets (prescription by a urologist, must be taught in the urologist's office)	Prostaglandin E, individually determined	Same as intracavernosal injections	Caution with anticoagulant use. Caution with history of priapism. Cardiology consult for history of arrhythmias, stroke, heart attack
Penile prosthesis	NA	Shorter penis	Risk of infection and need to re-implant

Women—Vaginal Comfort Aids

Treatment	Dose	Side Effects	Comments
Vaginal moisturizers	Twice weekly	NA	Water or silicon based, no glycerin
Vaginal lubricants	For sexual activity	Warming gels may produce a burning sensation	Water or silicon based, no glycerin
Estradiol vaginal inserts	10 micrograms, follow instructions	None	Should not be used if cancer is hormone-sensitive

Table 6.3 Continued

Women—Sexual Pleasure Aids

Treatment	Dose	Side Effects	Contraindications
Vibrators	To increase blood flow in erectile tissues, such as clitoris, vagina	NA	Enjoyable for foreplay or individual sexual activity
Clitoral pumps	To increase blood flow to clitoris	NA	Improves orgasmic function
Sexual Counseling			
Individual or couple sexual counseling	Spacing of sessions varies	NA	Usually addresses sex education (including use of sexual aids) and support
Individual sex therapy	Typically weekly sessions	NA	Addresses sex education, low sexual desire, performance anxiety, low confidence, grief regarding loss of sexual function, adjustment to illness-related sexual dysfunction
Couple sex therapy	Typically weekly or biweekly sessions	NA	Addresses sex education, desire discrepancy, coping with sexual dysfunction, couple conflict that interferes with sexual relationship, couple adjustment to illness-related sexual dysfunction

nonhormonally based medication shown to increase desire in premenopausal women, has been used off label with postmenopausal women and may be of value in the context of cancer.

Pelvic floor rehabilitation can address pain with orgasm for both men and women as it may relate to pelvic floor dysfunction. Women can learn vaginal dilation and muscle release. Men can strengthen their pelvic floor to support erectile function.

Biopsychosocial Clinical Management

Combining psychosocial and biomedical interventions is necessary to address all biopsychosocial aspects of sexuality after cancer treatment. Psychoeducation that includes information about sexual side effects, emotional responses, and relationship impacts as well as rehabilitation strategies should be offered to all patients before treatment starts. The depth of information must be tailored to each patient.

Biopsychosocial clinical management begins before treatment and follows treatment and includes the following:

- Partner presence whenever possible
- Addressing pretreatment expectations by providing education about the sexual side effects, rehabilitation, and emotional and couple adaptation
- Posttreatment offer of sexual aids to the man and to the partner as needed
- Posttreatment assessment of patient and partner psychological and couple adjustment
- Triaging support, based on clinical assessment to include monthly or three-monthly supportive counseling or ongoing, weekly or biweekly individual or couples sex therapy
- Attention to sexual orientation and cultural issues
- Coordination with other healthcare providers, such as urologists, radiation oncologists, medical oncologists, nurses, sexual medicine urologists, endocrinologists, primary care providers

When cancer treatment–related side effects emerge, biomedical interventions should always be offered in some combination with psychosocial interventions. Some patients will benefit simply by being educated about the sexual side effects of treatment and given guidance about what can be expected with respect to sexual recovery. Including the partner helps start the recovery of sexual intimacy from the same point and is beneficial for the relationship. If a patient has a close relationship with a partner or good social support, the work to develop a new sexual paradigm can proceed independently. Patients who are particularly distressed, have unrealistic expectations, or wish for closer monitoring because of lack of confidence will benefit from periodic visits with a clinician trained in relevant psychosexual counseling. Patients who are single and have concerns about future relationships may also need the support of a clinician, although the intensity of the support will depend on the assessment of the patient's ability to reflect on his or her needs, analyze potential situations, and maintain optimism versus pessimism about success. For some patients, sexual losses secondary to cancer treatment trigger preexisting mental illness or suicidal thoughts or plans. Those patients are best treated by a mental health professional. Patients who present with either preexisting relationship or sexual problems, or those whose sexual losses are so profound as to result in a deep grief reaction and despair, will need a more intensive follow-up via a referral to a psychosexual therapist who may treat the patient individually or with the partner.

Access to combined sexual health interventions provides patients with an opportunity to maximize sexual recovery after cancer treatment. Patients report that it can result in a richer, expanded sexual repertoire, deeper emotional closeness in their relationship, and greater sexual satisfaction despite the functional challenges.

Case Study

Mrs. G was a 53-year-old married woman who presented with her husband for couples sex therapy because sexual activity had become infrequent and unsatisfying since her treatment for her muscle-invasive bladder cancer 3 years prior to her evaluation. After her bladder was removed, the surgeon constructed a neobladder from her intestine. Mrs. G said that her new bladder was amazingly functional; she had no urinary problems at all. However, she had not been told that she would lose her uterus and her ovaries as part of her treatment, and after surgery she found herself in full-fledged, very symptomatic menopause. She said during the evaluation that she had always been somewhat shy about sex, but now she had pain with intercourse and was always angry when making love. Her husband confirmed this and said that he felt much compassion for her. From his vantage point, while he loved having sex with her, he wanted her to be happier and have sex because she wanted it, not for himself. They both said that they talked comfortably about these things together. Further evaluation determined that there were no issues in the relationship. However, when asked, Mrs. G acknowledged that she had not grieved her sexual function losses and that she was not aware of aids to sexual functioning that would make intercourse more comfortable. Although she had come for couples sex therapy, it was recommended that she engage in individual sex therapy to receive education about sexual aids and work through her grief about sexual losses. She accepted the recommendation and engaged fully in treatment. Later, she and her husband were seen together and were guided through sensate focus exercises as a way of comfortably returning to their sexual relationship.

Professional Issues and Service Implementation

Sexual health expertise is generally not available in usual care, and as a result sexual concerns are not addressed. According to the research literature, healthcare providers are not equipped to discuss sexual issues and tend to avoid them. In addition, patients are reluctant to bring up sexual issues because they are very personal and because they are uncertain whether such a discussion is legitimately an aspect of their cancer care. Finally, patients worry about making their healthcare providers uncomfortable.

How should sexual healthcare be routinely provided? While it is logically reasonable to have sexual health clinics that concentrate qualified providers, patients and healthcare providers tend to broach sexual issues more easily when sexual health care is embedded in a cancer survivorship program. From the patient's point of view, embedding sexual health experts in a survivorship program legitimizes those concerns. From the healthcare provider's point of view, a sexual health resource that is easily available supports patient-centered oncology care, obviates the challenge of finding a rare resource, and makes the conversation about sex easier.

Some countries have trained sex therapists. In the United States, the American Association of Sexuality Educators, Counselors and Therapists (aasect.org) certifies sex therapy counselors (usually nurses or physicians) and sex therapists (usually mental health providers) after extensive training and lists them by state on its website. The Society for Sex Therapy and Research (sstar.org) similarly lists sex therapists, but not all may be certified by AASECT. Many of these experts are in private practice, while some are attached to institutions. Reimbursement for services varies by country and by the healthcare system. In the United Kingdom, patients can look for a sex therapist in their local area on the website of the College of Sexual and Relationship Therapists (https://www.cosrt.org.uk), the Institute of Psychosexual Medicine (https://www.ipm.org.uk), or an organization called Relate (https://www.relate.org.uk/relationship-help/help-sex).

Oncology practitioners must become more familiar with human sexuality and with the sexual side effects of cancer and cancer treatments. Understanding these basic concepts would create more comfort for the necessary conversations and a better ability to refer patients to available resources. Oncology providers also must be aware of available resources for their own education and for patients. Three training opportunities for healthcare providers are (1) the University of Michigan Postgraduate Sexual Health Certificate Program (https://ssw.umich.edu/offices/continuing-education/certificate-courses/sexual-health); (2) Prostate Cancer Canada TrueNTH Clinician Training Program SHARe (https://truenth.ca/); and (3) Prostate Cancer UK TrueNTH Clinician Training Program "Talking about Sex" (https://talkingaboutsex-prostatecancer.org/).

These programs can be accessed and completed online. All have, in the past, included international trainees. The University of Michigan program requires at least one on-campus visit. It is a one-year program focused on sexuality in general, not only on sexuality and cancer, although cancer-related sexual issues are addressed.

The Prostate Cancer Canada program is more intensive; it available for a low fee and can be completed in nine sessions. The Prostate Cancer UK program is free and can be completed in 1 hour.

In the context of rare sexual health resources, telehealth has become a methodology for providing access to sexual health support for cancer patients. Leslie Schover, Ph.D., a long-term researcher in sexual health in cancer, developed the website Will2Love (https://www.will2love.com/) that provides, among other information, some strategies for symptom management and psychological coping. The Movember Foundation TrueNTH has supported the development of online psychosexual interventions in prostate cancer that are currently available online in Canada (SHARe clinic https://truenth.ca/) and the UK (Maximising Sexual Wellbeing https://prostate.lifeguidewebsites.org/player/play/prostate). A US TrueNTH intervention for prostate cancer patients and their partners will become available in 2020. These online resources are valuable as psychoeducational tools that can provide some degree of tailoring to individuals' needs. However, they do not substitute for a conversation about sexual concerns, support for loss and grief, and a nuanced approach to individuals' problems as they navigate sexual problems and sexual relationships during and after cancer treatment.

Regardless of immediately available resources, the management of sexual problems and sexual relationships requires that all those providing services to cancer patients are aware that sexual recovery after cancer requires a multidisciplinary approach. Sex therapists generally understand that in order to provide appropriate care, they must collaborate with members of other disciplines, especially with pelvic floor rehabilitation specialists, mental health providers, healthcare providers who manage chronic conditions, such as cancer, and others.

🔍 ***The challenge is to ensure that oncology care providers also recognize the need to have a database of relevant specialists to whom they can refer as needed.*** Providing sexual healthcare in oncology care remains an aspirational goal. However, setting out all the parameters for managing sexual health issues for individuals with cancer can lead to raising clinicians' awareness that all who care for cancer patients must work in concert and advocate for the inclusion of sexual health as a critical aspect of usual care in cancer.

References

1. Wettergren L, Kent EE, Mitchell SA, et al. Cancer negatively impacts on sexual function in adolescents and young adults: the AYA HOPE study. *Psychooncology* 2017;26(10):1632–1639.

2. Resnick MJ, Koyama T, Fan KH, et al. Long-term functional outcomes after treatment for localized prostate cancer. *N Engl J Med* 2013;368(5):436–445.

3. Reese JB, Handorf E, Haythornthwaite JA. Sexual quality of life, body image distress, and psychosocial outcomes in colorectal cancer: a longitudinal study. *Support Care Cancer* 2018;26(10):3431–3440.

4. Robinson PJ, Bell RJ, Christakis MK, et al. Aromatase inhibitors are associated with low sexual desire causing distress and fecal incontinence in women: an observational study. *J Sex Med* 2017;14(12):1566–1574.

5. Rhoten BA. Head and neck cancer and sexuality: a review of the literature. *Cancer Nurs* 2016;39(4):313–320.

6. Vroege JA, Gijs L, Hengeveld MW. Classification of sexual dysfunctions: towards DSM-V and ICD-11. *Compr Psychiatry* 1998;39(6):333–337.

7. McCabe MP, Sharlip ID, Lewis R, et al. Incidence and prevalence of sexual dysfunction in women and men: a consensus statement from the Fourth International Consultation on Sexual Medicine 2015. *J Sex Med* 2016;13(2):144–152.

8. Bober SL, Varela VS. Sexuality in adult cancer survivors: challenges and intervention. *J Clin Oncol* 2012;30(30):3712–3719.

9. Walker LM, Wassersug RJ, Robinson JW. Psychosocial perspectives on sexual recovery after prostate cancer treatment. *Nature Rev Urol* 2015;12(3):167–176.

10. Rosser BR, Capistrant B, Torres B, et al. The effects of radical prostatectomy on gay and bisexual men's mental health, sexual identity and relationships: qualitative results from the Restore Study. *Sex Relation Ther* 2016;31(4):446–461.

11. Tanner T, Galbraith M, Hays L. From a woman's perspective: life as a partner of a prostate cancer survivor. *J Midwifery Womens Health* 2011;56(2):154–160.

12. Gilbert E, Ussher JM, Hawkins Y. Accounts of disruptions to sexuality following cancer: the perspective of informal carers who are partners of a person with cancer. *Health* 2009;13(5):523–541.

13. Wittmann D, Northouse L, Crossley H, et al. A pilot study of potential preoperative barriers to couples' sexual recovery after radical prostatectomy for prostate cancer. *J Sex Marital Ther* 2014;41(2):155–168.

14. Gibson AW, Radix AE, Maingi S, Patel S. Cancer care in lesbian, gay, bisexual, transgender and queer populations. *Future Oncol* 2017;13(15):1333–1344.

15. Rosen RC, Riley A, Wagner G, et al. The International Index of Erectile Function (IIEF): a multidimensional scale for assessment of erectile dysfunction. *Urology* 1997;49(6):822–830.

16. Rosen R, Brown C, Heiman J, et al. The Female Sexual Function Index (FSFI): a multidimensional self-report instrument for the assessment of female sexual function. *J Sex Marital Ther* 2000;26(2):191–208.

17. Wei JT, Dunn RL, Litwin MS, et al. Development and validation of the Expanded Prostate Cancer Index composite (EPIC) for comprehensive assessment of health-related quality of life in men with prostate cancer. *Urology* 2000;56(6):899–905.

18. Gilbert SM, Dunn RL, Hollenbeck BK, et al. Development and validation of the Bladder Cancer Index: a comprehensive, disease specific measure of health related quality of life in patients with localized bladder cancer. *The Journal of urology.* 2010;183(5):1764–1769.

19. Cella D, Riley W, Stone A, et al. The Patient-Reported Outcomes Measurement Information System (PROMIS) developed and tested its first wave of adult self-reported health outcome item banks: 2005–2008. *J Clin Epidemiol* 2010;63(11):1179–1194.

20. Kroenke K, Spitzer RL, Williams JB. The PHQ-9: validity of a brief depression severity measure. *J Gen Intern Med* 2001;16(9):606–613.

21. Watson M, Grassi L. Recognizing and managing suicide risk. In Watson M, Kissane DW, eds. *Management of Clinical Depression and Anxiety* (Chapter 4). New York: Oxford University Press, 2017.

Further Reading

Brotto L, Barker M, eds. *Mindfulness in Sexual and Relationship Therapy*. Routledge Press, 2014.

This book is recommended as a manual for clinicians who wish to include mindfulness as a tool for helping patients increase sexual arousal.

Schover L. *Sexuality and Fertility After Cancer*. John Wiley & Sons, 1997.

This valuable primer on the issues that cancer patients face when their sexual function is affected by cancer and its treatment provides a hopeful yet realistic perspective as well as suggestions for maximizing sexual health in the context of cancer.

Ussher J, Perz J, Rosser SBR. *Gay and Bisexual Men Living with Prostate Cancer: From Diagnosis to Recovery*. Harrington Park Press LLC, 2018.

Despite its focus on prostate cancer, this book can help readers understanding how gay and bisexual men cope with the sexual side effects of cancer in general. The book summarizes up-to-date research and includes personal stories and clinical experiences.

Weiner L, Avery Clark C. *Sensate Focus in Sex Therapy: The Illustrated Manual*. Routledge Press, 2017.

This book is recommended because it not only describes in detail what sensate focus is and what it is not, it also offers step-by-step guidance for instructing patients how to use this method for increasing sexual comfort and intimacy.

Chapter 7

Couple Therapy for Sexual Dysfunction

Talia I. Zaider and David W. Kissane

Learning Objectives

After reading this chapter the clinician will be able to:

1. Recognize presentations of couple distress in cancer care
2. Have the confidence and skills needed to meet with couples and assess their support needs
3. Employ strategies that help couples communicate more openly about cancer and its care
4. Employ strategies that guide patients and their partners to plan successfully to meet their ongoing sexual health, fertility, and relationship needs
5. Employ strategies that help couples to sustain their positive life focus despite cancer

Background Evidence

A large body of literature has documented the challenges that arise for couples coping with cancer, as well as the relational processes that facilitate or impede individual adjustment. What emerges is an understanding of the patient and partner as an interconnected and mutually influencing system, evident in the concordant distress levels consistently found among cancer patients and their partners.

Risk Factors

Do the onset and the treatment of cancer endanger couple relationships? Despite the potential for severe strain on relationships resulting from intensive cancer treatment, the rates of divorce after a cancer diagnosis or treatment in one partner do not seem to differ from that in the general population.[1] Exceptions include young age, recent marriage, female gender, and difficult cancers that profoundly change functioning (e.g., brain tumors).

A recent study of approximately 2,000 young adult cancer survivors found significantly higher rates of divorce/separation compared to healthy controls.[2] In brain tumor patients, younger age and shorter marital duration were significant risk factors for divorce. Patient gender also plays a major role, with divorce or separation six times more likely to occur when the patient is female vs. male (20% vs. 3%).[3]

For couples who do remain together, is there evidence of increased marital distress resulting from cancer? Here the data vary, with many couples enjoying greater closeness following a diagnosis.[4] Prospective studies of couples coping with cancer have indicated that communication and marital satisfaction may decline over time, from diagnosis (a time of crisis and therefore increased cohesion) to subsequent phases in which couples may be more vulnerable to discord or loss of intimacy due to the cumulative effects of treatment.[5] As treatment-related complications become chronic, the long-term strain on couples becomes more pronounced.

Even among couples who remain together and report marital satisfaction, cancer treatment can distort communication and redefine relationship roles. When protective buffering inhibits open dialogue about cancer concerns, couples suffer worse psychosocial outcomes.[6] Sharing grief and distress is especially beneficial when partners perceive one another to respond in a supportive manner.[7]

When there is loss of sexual intimacy, couples will often shield one another from feelings of embarrassment or shame by withdrawing from physical contact altogether. In doing so, they avoid acknowledging even the most obvious physical changes due to surgery or hormone therapies. This can become a challenge in advanced cancer patients as well. A recent study of over 900 advanced cancer patients indicated that more than half had a strong desire for physical intimacy and felt their illness had impaired their ability to sustain sexual closeness.[8] Mutual avoidance confers greater risk of poor adjustment to such disruptions. Clinicians can model more direct communication by proactively asking patients and their partners about their physical relationship.

Which Relationship Factors Predict Individuals' Adjustment to Cancer?

The rationale for providing couple-based support in oncology is based on the need to restore and strengthen relationships and on the recognition that doing so protects the psychological adjustment of the individual patient and caregiver. Couples' communication patterns have been consistently predictive of individual distress, largely through their effect on intimacy.

One longitudinal study of breast cancer patients from initial diagnosis to 5 years afterward found that patients in distressed marriages had a slower recovery in distress levels, treatment side effects, and performance status. Similarly, a systematic review of dyadic studies in colorectal cancer concluded that relationship qualities (e.g., communication, support behaviors) significantly impacted patients' and partners' psychological adjustment to diagnosis and treatment.[9]

The extent to which couples manage cancer-related distress jointly, referred to as "we-ness" or "communal coping," has been consistently linked to better individual adjustment (e.g., self-efficacy, distress) as well as higher relationship functioning.[10] Finding ways to preserve or even amplify the identity and coping capacity of the couple as a unit is an important target for couple therapies.

Efficacy of Couple-Based Therapies in Oncology

At this early stage, the literature on couple-based interventions in oncology has not yet converged on a set of evidence-based best practices to guide clinicians but offers a diversity of approaches and targeted outcomes to consider. Some interventions enlist the partner as a coach or surrogate therapist in service of strengthening the patient's coping response, whereas others target specific relationship processes (e.g., communication) to enhance well-being for both partners. The couple-based interventions with empirical support are typically brief (six to eight visits) and draw from behavioral marital therapy techniques by focusing on enhancing communication or coping skills. Most interventions have been developed predominantly for couples facing breast[11] or prostate[12] cancers, as these illnesses directly impact sexual intimacy. Interventions for couples facing advanced cancer are sparser.

Over the past decade, meta-analyses have aggregated findings from randomized trials of couple interventions in cancer and have concluded that the benefits of this approach are significant but modest in magnitude.[13] Badr and Krebs (2013) found that across 20 randomized controlled trials, couple interventions had small but promising effects ($g = 0.21$–0.31) on physical and psychological quality-of-life outcomes for patients and partners. Another systematic review of couple-based interventions showed partial effectiveness, although differences in intervention content, study design, and measurement selection across studies limited interpretation.[14] A further meta-analysis of couple-based interventions across multiple chronic illnesses (e.g., cancer, cardiovascular disease, arthritis) found significant but small effects on depression, pain, and marital functioning.[15] In about half of the studies reviewed, patients receiving couple therapy improved significantly more on these outcomes relative to usual care or a patient-specific intervention.

Most of these trials offered therapy to all couples universally without triaging couples with greater need. Yet there is evidence that couple therapies are especially potent for patients or partners who have higher cancer-specific distress, poorer communication, or poorer marital quality. Clinicians can use brief assessment strategies (see the section on assessment principles below) to identify couples with greater psychosocial challenges who may benefit most from a specialized, relationship-based approach.

Summary of Background Evidence

Studies indicate that patients and their partners respond to cancer as an interconnected and mutually influencing system, with consistent evidence of concordant distress levels. Risk factors for marital separation or divorce following cancer diagnosis include younger age, more recently formed relationships, female gender, and more difficult cancers associated with behavioral changes (e.g., brain tumors). Relationship factors are strongly associated with the individual adjustment of patient or partner, including constructive communication with supportive response and joint or communal coping. Meta-analytic studies suggest significant but modest effects of couple-based interventions in oncology, with more recent evidence of increased benefit for patients and partners who present at baseline with higher distress, poorer communication, and/or poorer marital quality.

Presenting Problems

Couple therapy programs are not routinely available in most oncology settings, so the usual referral pathway (e.g., couple requesting marital therapy) may not apply. Instead, any oncology provider may decide to see a couple together for various reasons associated with illness management, whether or not there is significant relationship discord. It is helpful for clinicians to recognize presenting psychosocial or relationship problems that can be normalized as "part of the territory" of cancer, in addition to those that are unique to the couple's interaction pattern or history. Most couples will suffer some amount of strain in their relationship due to illness, the nature of which will be shaped by the specific treatment course, its chronicity, and any resulting disruptions to quality of life.

Reasons to consider conjoint sessions with a couple include the following:

- The patient's planned treatment or surgery is expected to cause significant family disruptions and caregiving demands.
- The couple is known to have conflictual interactions preceding the cancer diagnosis and therefore may be prone to exacerbations while coping with illness (e.g., couples with unresolved attachment injuries, or prior intentions to separate).
- Psychiatric care for the patient is at an impasse and added support is needed from an intimate partner.
- The patient's individual support needs are best addressed by involving the partner but there is concern about the partner's caregiving capacity, due to disengagement or history of psychiatric morbidity. In this case, conjoint meetings may be a means of drawing in a reluctant partner or facilitating his or her access to support.
- Disease progression brings end-of-life discussions to the fore, prompting greater involvement of loved ones in patient care.

Regardless of the impetus for conjoint meetings, couples often experience one or more of the cancer-related challenges listed below. Explicitly acknowledging these challenges as normal in this context can provide great relief to couples, who otherwise misattribute their experience of disruption to their own or their partners' inadequacies.

Role Challenges

From initial diagnosis onward, couples find their roles quickly redefined by the demands of the medical crisis at hand. Healthcare systems further reinforce the designation of "patient" versus "caregiver," a distinction that carries implications for how decisions are made, who is privy to what information, and to whom psychosocial support is targeted. On this basis alone, couples often experience a loss of mutuality and "we-ness" that disrupts the natural rhythm of their daily lives. Couples for whom these role shifts are problematic will describe cancer as having a divisive or separating effect.

For some couples, distance grows as the "caregiver" partner infers that his or her job is to be protected at all costs, to avoid burdening the patient and to manage stress independently. Patients in turn experience the loss of their sense of self as well as loss of a contributing, care-providing partner in the relationship. Role challenges also include dilemmas about who oversees what aspects of cancer management (e.g., scheduling appointments, checking medication lists, communicating concerns to providers, advocating).

Decisions about the distribution of these tasks can cause friction in couples who historically struggle with conflict around control and responsibility. An additional manifestation of role challenges occurs when each partner adopts a rigid and polarized stance regarding an uncertain prognosis. Those determined to preserve hope may complain that their partner is too negative or pessimistic. Those more preoccupied with fears of recurrence or disease progression may complain that their partner is dismissive and minimizing. As couples divide the "emotional labor" of coping with cancer, the polarization of these roles leads to conflict about who is "right" as opposed to appreciating the value of holding both perspectives.

Transition Challenges

John Rolland, in his family systems illness model, elegantly maps out the psychosocial challenges associated with phase and course of illness. Couples may present with difficulties transitioning from active treatment to survivorship: Partners may differ in their eagerness to restore normality and "reset" to precancer expectations, even when treatment-related symptoms have not entirely abated. Another manifestation of this challenge is the couple who persists in their vigilance for signs and symptoms of cancer well past its utility. Couples transitioning from acute to chronic phases of illness, with an indefinite but routine treatment course ahead, sometimes find that one or both partners remain in "crisis mode" when this coping style is no longer congruent with their illness phase. The increased length of survival for many with advanced cancer presents unique challenges for couples, who must remain vigilant and prepared on some level, but also avoid burning out, or grieving prematurely. The saying "don't leave before you leave" becomes a central concern for couples who are aware of a limited future, but for whom loss is by no means imminent.

Communication Challenges

Holding back concerns about prognosis, limiting what is safe to talk about, or keeping secrets about illness in the family are common challenges experienced by couples, as many subscribe to the widespread belief that "talking about it makes it worse." Couples experience this same behavior in their social network, as friends and relatives struggle to respond skillfully to their experience with illness. Couples can find it especially difficult to talk about changes in functioning or appearance following treatment, in the service of avoiding embarrassment. The behaviors and interactions that develop over time to support this avoidance (e.g., withdrawing from sexual activity, reducing social engagements) can have the effect of gradually diminishing a couple's capacity for pleasure and meaningful activity, thereby amplifying the sense of loss accompanying these changes.

Conflict/Anger Challenges

Conflict can manifest when longstanding fractures in the relationship become magnified under the strain of cancer diagnosis and treatment. Unresolved emotional injuries (e.g., infidelity, loyalty binds, blaming/critical communication patterns) emerge, causing resentment for the partner or guilt for the patient. Normative anger as an expression of the grief and unfairness felt by patients and their partners, who "didn't sign up for this," can also be a powerful undercurrent in the relationship, driving couples to bicker more often about seemingly minor issues. Clinicians can normalize and acknowledge the legitimacy of anger as a shared response to illness. Finally, anger can arise when one partner implicitly blames the other for the cancer diagnosis itself, particularly when there has been a history of health risk behaviors (e.g., smoking, alcohol misuse, substance dependence). Partners can become tirelessly consumed with managing the patient's health behavior, unaware that their tendency to overfunction in this regard invites passivity and inertia on the part of the patient.

Boundary Challenges

A common task for couples following a cancer diagnosis is to negotiate boundaries with extended family and friends. Many couples benefit from the involvement of a family "navigator," such as a family member or friend whose professional or personal experience lends important knowledge about interfacing with healthcare systems or accessing resources. Yet the sudden and intensified involvement of "outside helpers" can have a diluting effect on the cohesiveness of the couple, as the family unit expands to accommodate the need for broader support. These boundary challenges frequently arise for younger couples, blended families, or couples early in their relationship formation. A cancer diagnosis can precipitate a young adult's regression to the care of a parent, or may prompt the need for increased support as extended family move in to help care for children, or join the patient at medical appointments, and thus in decision-making. In a blended family, adult children may step in to take charge of care for an elderly parent, excluding a newer stepparent. Couples are thus challenged to preserve their sense of agency as they delegate and maintain control over who has "membership" in the patient's unit of care, and dilemmas about who is entitled to be "in" or "out" of this group can generate considerable conflict in couples.

The converse of this is the couple that is isolated and in need of "parenting" but disengaged/estranged from extended family. Separated couples may re-engage for support, yet with ambivalence and an uncertain sense of responsibility.

Intimacy Challenges

Changes in physical appearance and/or sexual functioning due to cancer treatment can easily disrupt the frequency and satisfaction with sexual intimacy in couples. Couples will rarely voice these concerns until asked, but often appreciate the opportunity to acknowledge the loss of a spontaneous physical relationship. These challenges can manifest as complaints of withdrawal from physical affection, reduced engagement with one another physically, and/or body image concerns and repulsion or fears about attractiveness to a well partner. Shame about either the presence or absence of sexual desire can limit communication about this issue, which further compounds the loss felt by couples as they tacitly agree to succumb to a sexless relationship.

Key Predicaments

Key predicaments contributing to these couple presentations are as follows:

1. Cancer-related
   a. Poor health literacy about cancer
   b. Poor understanding of prognosis and goals of care provision
   c. Breaks in continuity of professional care in public settings
   d. Limited relationship with clinician
   e. Complex disease and treatment aspects beyond the usual
2. Couple-related
   a. Couple do not attend oncology consultations together
   b. Skewed styles in gaining information about cancer
   c. Different coping approaches to deal with the stress of the diagnosis
   d. Variant preferences for treatment approach
   e. Particular religious beliefs impacting treatment choices
3. System-related
   a. Engaged with public versus private healthcare system
   b. Financial strain due to factors beyond the couple
   c. Geographic or access issues
   d. Language or ethnic issues
   e. Religious or moral differences with the treating institution

Assessment Principles for Couple Dimensions of Care

The following principles guide the assessment process used to define couple concerns, to understand who they are and what dynamics appear prominent, and to help them reach agreement about the goals of psychosocial care that may follow this assessment.

1. *Who should be invited to an initial meeting? Who is the unit of care?* Consider an initial assessment of the presenting patient and a follow-up assessment of the couple when this appears indicated. If the couple presents together in the waiting room for a psychosocial assessment appointment, ask the patient directly if he or she wishes to be seen alone or with the partner. If the couple expresses some difference in perspective (e.g., partner wishes to join the patient, but patient wishes to be seen alone), the clinician can suggest seeing the patient for the first half of the appointment and bringing the partner in for the last 10 to 15 minutes for a joint discussion. Consider their preferences. When the

referral letter identifies a specific couple reason for assessment, this may guide the clinician's choice in starting immediately with the couple.

2. **Balance assessment of individual versus relational support needs.** It is important to assess each individual to ascertain (i) understanding of clinical predicament; (ii) coping response; (iii) family background, support base, and dynamics; and (iv) individual risk factors for psychiatric, relational, or sexual disorder. An assessment of the couple is also vital to ascertain (i) relational history; (ii) relational events; (iii) stresses on the couple historically and currently; and (iv) perception of current needs and concerns.

3. **Elicit key agenda items for couple.** The creation of an agreed agenda early in the session allows for prioritizing issues or concerns and eventually establishing a timeline for addressing relevant concerns.

4. **Listen to the couple's illness story.** Listening to the narrative of illness diagnosis and early decision-making reveals the emotional response to the cancer and may expose the pattern of mutual support or early couple difficulties.

5. **Ask the couple how they met.** Develop an understanding of the strengths of the relationship through the story of initial meeting and attraction. What is the rhythm of their relationship? Any challenges?

6. **Create a genogram.** The family tree for each partner tells much about family patterns of relating; dealing with loss, illness, and death; and sources of strength and vulnerability.

7. **Assess the impact of cancer on the relationship, and elicit each partner's perception of self and other coping.** A circular exploration of the impact of cancer on each party and their coping and concerns begins to allow for mutual empathic support to be expressed by each partner, with time for confirmation by the other of accuracy of the distress and coping perceived.

8. **Ask proactively about sexual intimacy.** Make explicit the nature, frequency, and style of both couple intimacy and coital interaction. What concerns and challenges are revealed?

9. **Assess the couple's communication style.** Examine communication patterns for the couple, including both strengths and barriers. What is talked about and with whom? What topics are off limits?

10. **Identify the couple's strengths and resources.** By summarizing the evident strengths of the relationship, you create a focus on pathways toward healing and gain, while avoiding too critical a focus on deficits.

11. **Formulate specific goals for therapy.** Agreeing on a small number of goals or targets to work on establishes a clear agenda and focus for ongoing work. Goals should be prioritized, taking easier issues first to create early progress ahead of tougher issues that will need time.

⚠️ Confounding challenges to watch for during assessment are as follows:

1. Pre-existing relational deficits—infidelity, separations, emotional withdrawal
2. High level of conflict—domestic violence, alcohol or drug abuse
3. Misunderstanding of cancer stage, seriousness, treatment goals or prognosis
4. Age of children—stress in young family with existential fears
5. Confounding mental illness in one party—unrecognized anxiety or depressive disorder
6. Couple isolation with few supports—childless couple, recent geographic moves
7. Migrant, refugee, ethnic barriers to care—language, health models, ethnic approach to illness and its treatment
8. Socioeconomic challenges—unemployment, rental instability, insurance and health access to care provision

Case Study

Complex relationship challenges emerged when a man lost his eye to cancer treatment. After a period of anosmia and then drooping of his left eyelid, a 45-year-old married father of two had his left eye enucleated as part of the management of a rare sinus tumor 4 years ago. Surgery was followed by radiation and chemotherapy, with an overall 70% survival prospect. He disliked wearing an eye patch, and radiation therapy had reduced the prospects of plastic surgery reconstruction. His disfigurement limited prior working roles in theater and the arts. He felt awkward, uncomfortable, unattractive, and unwelcome at group events. Children stared at him, and he retreated to the side of groups rather than require others to have to relate to him.

He had found his wife resentful at his social withdrawal and intermittent fatigue, associated with his cancer survivorship. He found it hard to provide as much care for their 10- and 4-year-old children as she wanted, and he was concerned about the safety of driving with a single eye. His wife had been depressed and undoubtedly very frightened by his cancer and its threat. She told him that she had considered divorce. They had pursued couples counseling, initially with a female therapist who promoted the strengths of their relationship, and then with a male counselor who focused more on the negatives. Progress was limited and he felt trapped.

He described his wife as angry and less loving, with a low level of libido, as a result of which he perceived that she rationed sexuality. He found sex to be healing and acknowledged yearning for this, carrying sexual fantasies that he be actively desired. The couple averaged coitus every 6 weeks, and after any fight, he felt despondent and thought about suicide as an escape.

He started seeing a psychologist individually, enjoying talking to a woman and appreciating her support. They developed goals, including work on both his inner sense of self and his marital relationship to help him move into a better emotional space and bring more fulfilment into his life. He needed to adopt a less critical stance toward his wife, using a courtship approach toward her rather than a sense of the entitlement of periodic sexual release. As he started to date her, express kindness, and offer reassurance about his survival, her mood lifted and their sense of mutual support grew. Joint activities with their children further increased harmony. All of this helped his self-esteem and what he could contribute to his family. Rather than his more entitled stance, fostering relational harmony saw a natural return to a more sexually fulfilling relationship without a formal therapeutic focus on this.

Investigations for Key Differential Diagnosis

Key Differentials

- Unrecognized psychiatric disorder in one partner
- Misunderstanding of cancer seriousness and treatment model
- Socioeconomic, cultural, or language barrier issues
- Undeclared drug and alcohol abuse, domestic violence, infidelity
- Stress over disabled or ill child with high care needs
- Cumulative illness in the family

Screening Measures That Could Be Useful

- Screen for depression: 9-item PHQ-9 questionnaire for major depression
- Screen for anxiety: 7-item GAD-7 questionnaire for anxiety disorder
- Screen for relational functioning: 12-item Family Relationships Index for relational patterns of communication, conflict resolution, and cohesion or teamwork
- Screen for marital distress: 7-item Dyadic Adjustment Scale

Additional Issues to Identify

- History of domestic violence or aggression
- Psychiatric history of partner/caregiver
- Concerns about children/adolescents who may be symptomatic and require specialized support
- Need for additional individual therapy/medication management
- Concerns about communication with primary oncology team, issues to facilitate/advocate on behalf of couple (e.g., multidisciplinary family meetings, informational needs, difficulties with symptom management). Who is the family's point person? Trusted contact in the care team?

Clinical Management

The flowchart in Figure 7.1 outlines potential paths of assessment and treatment of couples.

- Clarify referral-on details.
- Specify the range of treatment options with reasons for choices.

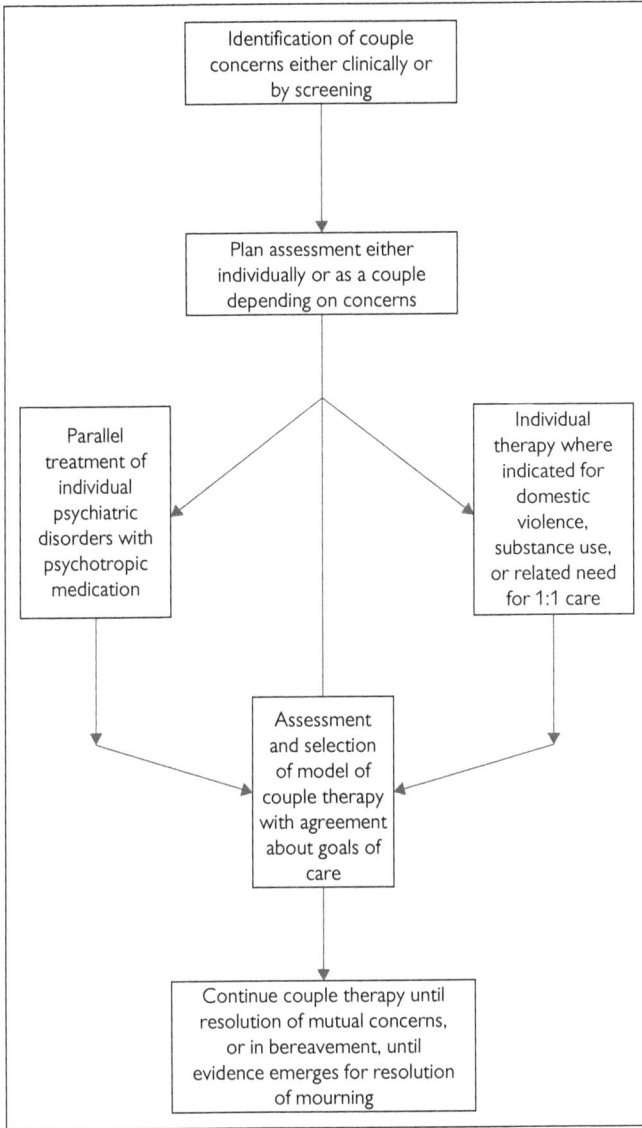

Figure 7.1 Flowchart outlining assessment and management of couple concerns in cancer care

- Specify systemic and other allied health features of management.
- Where pharmacotherapy is advised, tabulate schedule of dose titration and key drug interactions. List consequential drug side effects to monitor.
- Specify key psychotherapeutic approaches as appropriate.

Couple Therapy

Early Stage/Survivorship Approaches to Therapy

Models of psychotherapy developed and tested for patients with early stage disease, or for those transitioning out of active treatment, aim to strengthen the couple's communication, joint problem-solving, and coping skills. Most of the techniques used in couple-based therapies for early stage cancers draw from behavioral marital therapy, with content specifically adapted to address cancer-related concerns. In most research trials, these types of interventions were tested with all couples facing a given cancer diagnosis, regardless of their level of distress or relational discord. As mentioned earlier, despite the modest efficacy of these interventions, there are data suggesting that these approaches may be especially beneficial for couples who begin therapy with more cancer-related concerns, higher distress, or worse communication and relationship quality. Clinicians may wish to target these higher-risk couples for greater effect.

The following components are commonly included.

Taking Stock of Cancer-Related Impact

Both as an assessment and intervention tool, clinicians are encouraged to invite the couple to discuss the impact of cancer on each of them individually, as well as on the relationship. This discussion is often the first opportunity for the couple to jointly reflect on before/after changes, particularly as they pertain to their ways of relating with one another. Circular questions can be used to elicit perceptions of cancer impact on the other as well as self. This questioning style tests partners' capacity for empathic attunement, encourages perspective taking, and stimulates dialogue between them as they become aware of differences and similarities in their perspectives.

Revising Definitions of Intimacy and Normalizing Feelings

A central task for couples coping with treatment-related changes in functioning or appearance, is to re-examine sources of intimacy in their relationship after the cancer diagnosis. Clinicians can offer an expanded notion of what constitutes intimacy, distinguishing between emotional and physical domains. Understanding what gestures of intimacy are most appreciated by each partner, and helping the couple articulate this openly, creates an opportunity to recognize the range of choices available to them. Couples may need strong encouragement to experiment with a more proactive and intentional approach to creating intimacy, a strategy that can be perceived at first as artificial. Home exercises such as sensate focus, planned date nights and rituals, or Suzanne Iasenza's (2011) "sexual menu" can be suggested as a means of guiding this process. John Gottman's notion of reciprocal bidding (i.e., attempts to turn toward one another for affection, attention, or positive connection) can be a helpful notion as couples are encouraged to be alert and responsive to their partners' idiosyncratic bids for connection.

Clinician flexibility is key, as one or both partners may resist a prescriptive approach. If partners protest the need to plan or structure intimate activity, the clinician should acknowledge the loss of spontaneity due to cancer and explore its meaning for each partner.

⚠ **In general, clinicians may need to normalize and open up dialogue about feelings of loss and shame, particularly around changes in sexual functioning. When they go unacknowledged and unexpressed, these feelings can powerfully shape relational behavior (e.g., withdrawal, irritability).**

Normalizing and helping couples talk openly about these feelings helps to counter negative assumptions partners develop about one another (e.g., "he is no longer attracted to me" vs. "he is embarrassed about his erectile dysfunction"). Clinicians emphasize the chance for discovery, creativity, risk taking, and play, relieving couples of the pressure to conform to old models of intimacy. For example, when the partner who previously initiated physical contact suffers a loss of libido, the well partner may take on this role. In the same vein, couples are encouraged to recognize that in the absence of desire or physiologic arousal, "willingness" can be a sufficient source of drive.

Strengthening Communication Skills

Couples struggling to communicate about treatment-related concerns and changes often appreciate guidance on how to do so safely and productively. Clinicians can initially observe a couple's communication patterns by **asking them to converse about topics of concern, or taking note in session of any cautiousness in expressing thoughts or feelings** and tendencies to interrupt or resort to criticism, blame, defensiveness, or withdrawal. **Feedback to couples about these observed patterns** serves as a basis for offering more constructive communication strategies. Clinicians may need to be quite active in session, setting limits on maladaptive behaviors and coaching partners to express themselves in ways that maximize the chances that they will be heard. **Chaotic and conflict-prone couples will benefit most from a structured, "speaker–listener" or turn-taking approach, as establishing ground rules for communication will provide needed safety to explore cancer-related concerns.** On the other hand, protectiveness is normalized as a common, cancer-induced threat to intimate communication. Rather than insist unilaterally that more talk is always better, clinicians do better to help couples reflect together on when and how disclosure of negative feelings (e.g., grief, fear) is constructive. Partners are encouraged to articulate and check any constraining beliefs, including concerns about burdening a partner with distress, about the helpfulness versus harm of crying together, and about the perceived pressure to reassure or problem solve in response to such disclosure.

Advanced Cancer Approaches and Bereavement Care

Models of therapy discussed here include emotion-focused and existentially oriented couple therapy, intimacy-enhancing couple therapy, and meaning-centered couple therapy, with extension of each of these models into bereavement care for the surviving partner.

Emotion-Focused and Existentially Oriented Couple Therapy

This is the most basic and essential model of psychotherapeutic care in the setting of advanced cancer and hospice care. Several key strategies form the bedrock of the model of care.

Naming and Normalizing Grief
As disease recurs and the diagnosis of advanced cancer is used, grief becomes prominent for the couple, who reveal tearful eyes at most consultations. Grief should be normalized as comprehensible, adaptive, and helpful when shared, for this typically fosters deeper closeness for the couple. Depending on the prognosis, discussion of the benefit or burden of anticipatory grief proves helpful to many, lest they get stuck in their grief.

Discussing Death and Dying
Just as naming grief is orienting for many, so too is direct discussion of death anxiety, with open use of the word "dying." If any doubt exists, permission can be sought to talk about dying when the clinician judges that such conversation is timely. Many seek to understand and be reassured about what will happen as the process of dying unfolds.

Diagnosing Dying
Palliative care services can do much to ameliorate this journey. Even helping the couple to recognize when dying has commenced can be an invaluable service to them.

Identifying Supportive Processes
The unfamiliarity of the modern couple with death and dying causes many to feel lost about what to do. Discussion of a roadmap of relevant activities and tasks can prove very helpful. Have they discussed and completed an advance care plan and last will and testament, appointed a healthcare proxy, and put their affairs in order? Have they discussed preferred place of dying? Are there pragmatic services and supports that would prove helpful to achieving their goals?

Living Life Until It Stops

The existential solution to the challenge of a finite life is not to focus on illness and frailty bringing sadness, but rather to stay in the present, attending to whoever is there, thus sustaining the role as spouse or parent. Lest the principle of "live in the moment" appears as another euphemism, it merits translation into real-time examples for the patient or couple at hand.

Talking About Goodbyes

For many, beyond these basic practicalities, talking about the process of saying goodbye proves helpful. Rather than being thought of as a final hug, reminiscing about the life shared together and its highlights, looking at photographs, reviewing accomplishments, recalling poignant memories, and discussing future hopes for the surviving partner are all worthwhile. Many go on to plan the funeral. Such talk is immensely helpful for the bereaved. Clinicians can affirm the courage involved when couples can share these intimate conversations.

One simple model of communication that can be encouraged involves the key headings of "I love you," "Please forgive me," "I forgive you," and "Goodbye." When children are involved, further principles include affirmation, through a statement of what the parent is "proud of" in the child, clarification that the parent does not want to die and regrets the onset of this illness, and acknowledgement that the parent wants his or her values and love to accompany the child into the future. Encourage children to ask themselves, "What would Mom want for me in this situation?" The notion of the parent becoming a guardian angel watching over the child can be helpful if culturally appropriate.

Intimacy-Enhancing Couple Therapy

Advanced illness typically brings as part of its burden the loss of libido, sexual arousal, and capacity for coitus. Couples may feel this loss yet struggle to acknowledge it openly. The concept of intimacy is often immediately apparent to the woman as important, her sexuality having been process-oriented throughout her life. When male sexuality is more outcome-oriented, with a focus on orgasm, discussion of the value of intimacy and its nature and practice can be crucial. This leads naturally to inviting conversation about what the couple can share in the remaining time and their priorities, opportunities, hopes, and wishes. Some simple techniques can make this explicit.

Normalizing Affection and Intimate Contact

Remove any awkwardness about touch and affection in hospital and public settings. Invite conversation about letting the illness draw the couple closer, mutually supporting and responding to each other's needs. Is there a place for massage? For sensate focus, stage 1 "petting"? Will the partner stay overnight in the inpatient setting?

Developing Priorities Through Hypothetical Timeline Planning

Invite the couple to each record individually their goals and wishes if life were sustained for three possible lengths of time—weeks to live, versus months, versus years. Have them share each other's lists and understand respective choices, leading to a shared plan for whatever life remains. This homework exercise often shifts priorities and fosters more open communication about a finite time, maximizing its use for the couple.

Reviewing and Recollecting

With a focus on the most intimate aspects of their relationship, invite them to privately reminisce about the joys and triumphs of their companionship, creating the means to celebrate and appreciate the relationship they have shared. Love, gratitude, forgiveness, and mutual appreciation can be fostered in this shared space.

Defining Their Legacy

Most couples leave a legacy. Individual therapies often focus on the patient and the life he or she has lived, with a relative neglect of the couple. By inviting them to consider their shared legacy, emphasis is returned to relational strengths, values, and accomplishments. Deepening awareness of their mutual successes enhances their joy and allows the possibility of acceptance of death, albeit with shared sadness at the closure of their relationship. Attention is naturally drawn to the future of the surviving partner, with permission hopefully being given to live life out fully and well.

Saying Goodbye

This most intimate of processes can be readily avoided, sometimes with regret in bereavement about the things left unsaid. On the other hand, a deeply connected and intimate couple will gain deep solace from completion of this courageous process, a celebration of their love and devotion to one another.

Meaning-Centered Couple Therapy

One particular development of existentially oriented therapy in the setting of advanced cancer is to place emphasis on optimizing the meaning and purpose of any time that remains.

⚠ **This has merit to counter the tendency of a person struggling with disease progression, symptom burden, and hopelessness to question the point of continued existence and to give up prematurely on life.**

A systematic review of studies of demoralization showed a prevalence of 15% in the palliative care setting, where pointlessness, helplessness, and hopelessness predominated, without necessarily developing into clinical depression. Recent randomized controlled trials of meaning-centered therapy, whether the Managing Cancer and Living Meaningfully (CALM) version[16] developed in Toronto or the adaptation of Victor Frankl's model[17] trialed in New York, showed benefits in sustaining morale and appreciation of the value of life. For patients exhibiting high levels of death anxiety at baseline and receiving CALM therapy, levels of demoralization were significantly reduced ($d = .51$).[18]

Because so much of life's meaning is found in the relational domain, meaning-centered therapy is very easily adapted to couples. The couple is asked to review the role they fulfill as a spouse and parent, often rating this family domain as one of the substantial sources of meaning and sustained purpose in their remaining life. Illness can preoccupy patients with bodily concerns, and the therapist can help to refocus attention on loved ones around them, helping them to see the value in their continuing role as a partner or relative.[19]

Bereavement Support

If the clinician has worked with a couple in palliative care, continuity is readily sustained for the surviving partner in bereavement. This can be especially valuable for those with strong bonds of attachment, who may have given so much to their caregiving role that the gap after death of their partner creates a deep emptiness. Complications such as clinical depression or prolonged grief disorder are readily treated, and the common model of support involves 6 to 10 sessions over 12 to 18 months, with early sessions held every 3 to 4 weeks and later sessions gradually moved to every 2 to 3 months until a satisfactory adaptation has been made. Direct knowledge of the deceased is invaluable to such care provision compared to grief counselors who only meet the bereaved after the death.

Professional Issues and Service Implementation

Policies

- As soon as children are involved, professional bodies immediately recognize the principle of family-centered care informing clinical practice. The International Association of Hospice and Palliative Care has long included the needs of caregivers and family as core components of practice, thus ensuring that patients and partners remain a genuine focus of clinical care.
- Most oncology consultations have partners or relatives attending with patients, pointing to their expectation for couple or family-centered care.

Recording and Communicating

- Documentation of these consultations is a basic responsibility.
- Inpatient medical records must document details of family meetings.
- More formal couple therapy is usually dealt with at an outpatient level.
- Correspondence back to the referring primary care practitioner is desirable to keep him or her informed of couple and family issues.

Legal Responsibilities

- Whenever issues exist at the couple or family level, a duty of care requires the clinician to refer appropriately for couple or family therapy.
- Encourage patients to put their affairs in order early in the journey of cancer treatment, including wills, power of attorney, healthcare directives, and attention to the care needs of children.

Common Ethical Dilemmas

- When seeing a couple, the therapist adopts a neutral stance with the goal of avoiding being drawn into an alliance with one party that might limit the trust and responsiveness of the other. Reflective comments might highlight the dilemma for the couple when tensions exist between them about what to do, thus locating responsibility for any choice as remaining with the couple.
- Sometimes, and more so in the family setting, competing needs become very apparent. Practical issues like discussion of respite care exemplify this dilemma well.

Teams and Supervision

- The multidisciplinary care team brings together clinicians with differing levels of training and expertise, especially across allied health domains. Couple and family behaviors will be noted at such team meetings, as goals of care are developed both for the patient and for the caregivers and family.
- The co-therapy model is an excellent means to build experience within teams and train less experienced clinicians in systemic approaches to care.
- Supervision of couple and family therapists can use a peer-group model to draw out diverse perspectives about coping and functioning, as well as to develop hypotheses and strategies about optimal ways to help.
- Comprehensive cancer centers that operate a couple and family clinic will usually have a supervisory process routinely functioning in the background so that less experienced staff members are gradually trained and supported in the work they do.

References

1. Laitala VS, Saarto T, Einiö EK, et al. Early-stage breast cancer is not associated with the risk of marital dissolution in a large prospective study of women. *Br J Cancer* 2015;113(3):543–437. doi:10.1038/bjc.2015.216

2. Kirchhoff AC, Yi J, Wright J, et al. Marriage and divorce among young adult cancer survivors. *J Cancer Surviv* 2012; 6(4):441–450. doi:10.1007/s11764-012-0238-6

3. Karraker A, Latham K. In sickness and in health? Physical illness as a risk factor for marital dissolution in later life. *J Health Soc Behav* 2015;56(3):420–435. doi:10.1177/0022146515596354

4. Drabe N, Wittmann L, Zwahlen D, et al. Changes in close relationships between cancer patients and their partners. *Psychooncology* 2013;22(6):1344–1352. doi:10.1002/pon.3144

5. Langer SL, Yi JC, Storer BE, Syrjala KL. Marital adjustment, satisfaction and dissolution among hematopoietic stem cell transplant patients and spouses: a prospective, five-year longitudinal investigation. *Psychooncology* 2010;19(2):190–200. doi:10.1002/pon.1542

6. Regan TW, Lambert SD, Kelly B, et al. Couples coping with cancer: exploration of theoretical frameworks from dyadic studies. *Psychooncology* 2015;24(12):1605–1617. doi:10.1002/pon.3854

7. Manne SL, Kashy DA, Kissane DW, et al. The course and predictors of perceived unsupportive responses by family and friends among women newly diagnosed with gynecological cancers. *Transl Behav Med* 2018 [E-pub before print]. doi:10.1093/tbm/iby087

8. Bond CB, Jensen PT, Groenvold M, Johnsen AT. Prevalence and possible predictors of sexual dysfunction and self-reported needs related to the sexual life of advanced cancer patients. *Acta Oncol* 2019;58(5):769–775. doi:10.1080/0284186X.2019.1566774

9. Kayser K, Acquati C, Reese JB, et al. A systematic review of dyadic studies examining relationship quality in couples facing colorectal cancer together. *Psychooncology* 2018;27(1):13–21. doi:10.1002/pon.4339

10. Traa MJ, Braeken J, De Vries J, et al. Sexual, marital, and general life functioning in couples coping with colorectal cancer: a dyadic study across time. *Psychooncology* 2015;24(9):1181–1188. doi:10.1002/pon.3801

11. Carroll AJ, Baron SR, Carroll RA. Couple-based treatment for sexual problems following breast cancer: a review and synthesis of the literature. *Support Care Cancer* 2016;24(8):3651–3659. doi:10.1007/s00520-016-3218-y

12. Manne SL, Kashy DA, Zaider T, et al. Couple-focused interventions for men with localized prostate cancer and their spouses: a randomized clinical trial. *Br J Health Psychol* 2019;24(2):396–418. doi:10.1111/bjhp.12359.

13. Badr H, Krebs P. A systematic review and meta-analysis of psychosocial interventions for couples coping with cancer. *Psychooncology* 2013;22(8):1688–1704. doi:10.1002/pon.3200

14. Baik OM, Adams KB. Improving the well-being of couples facing cancer: a review of couples-based psychosocial interventions. *J Marital Fam Ther* 2011;37(2):250–266. doi:10.1111/j.1752-0606.2010.00217.x

15. Martire LM, Schulz R, Helgeson VS, et al. Review and meta-analysis of couple-oriented interventions for chronic illness. *Ann Behav Med* 2010;40(3):325–342. doi:10.1007/s12160-010-9216-2

16. Rodin G, Lo C, Rydall A, et al. Managing Cancer and Living Meaningfully (CALM): a randomized controlled trial of a psychological intervention for patients with advanced cancer. *J Clin Oncol* 2018;36(23):2422–2432. doi:10.1200/JCO.2017.77.1097

17. Breitbart W, Pessin H, Rosenfeld B, et al. Individual meaning-centered psychotherapy for the treatment of psychological and existential distress: a randomized controlled trial in patients with advanced cancer. *Cancer* 2018;124(15):3231–3239. doi:10.1002/cncr.31539

18. An E, Lo C, Hales S, et al. Demoralization and death anxiety in advanced cancer. *Psychooncology* 2018;27(11):2566–2572. doi:10.1002/pon.4843

19. Lethborg C, Kissane DW, Schofield P. Meaning and Purpose (MaP) therapy, I: therapeutic processes and themes in advanced cancer. *Palliat Support Care* 2019;17(1):13–20. doi:10.1017/S1478951518000871

Further Reading

Greenberg LS, Johnson SM. *Emotionally Focused Therapy for Couples*. New York: Guilford Press, 2010.

Generic, classic clinical guide to couple therapy, but not in the setting of cancer. Many case examples.

Kissane DW, Bloch S. *Family-Focused Grief Therapy: A Model of Family-Centred Care Curing Palliative Care and Bereavement.* Buckingham, UK: Open University Press, 2002 (reprinted 2008).

Replete with clinical examples of approaches to family-centered care.

Kissane DW, Parnes F, eds. *Bereavement Care for Families.* New York: Routledge, 2014.

Multiauthored volume on approaches to family care from psycho-oncology through bereavement.

Zaider TI, Kissane DW. Couples therapy in advanced cancer: using intimacy and meaning to reduce existential distress. Chapter 14 in Watson M, Kissane DW, eds, *Handbook of Psychotherapy in Cancer Care.* Chichester, UK: Wiley-Blackwell, 2011.

Clinically oriented chapter describing techniques and strategies for couple care in oncology.

Zaider TI, Kissane DW. Psychosocial interventions for couples and families coping with cancer. Chapter 69 in Holland J, Breitbart WS, Butow P, et al., eds., *Psycho-Oncology*, 3rd ed. New York: Oxford University Press, 2015: 526–531.

Systemic care provision described in the comprehensive psycho-oncology text.

Index

Tables, figures and boxes are indicated by *t*, *f* and *b* following the page number

For the benefit of digital users, indexed terms that span two pages (e.g., 52–53) may, on occasion, appear on only one of those pages.

abdomino-perineal resection surgery, 22t
adolescents, and young adults
 age and maturity, ethical dilemmas, 92–94
 assessment, 72–76
 background of, 63–68
 body image, 68–69, 74
 cancer treatment, indirect effects on sexual health, 69b
 care team communication and records, 90–91
 care team policy, training, and supervision, 94–95
 childhood cancer survivors, 64–65
 clinical management, 77–89
 clinical practice guidelines, 66–68
 cognitive-behavioral therapy, 83
 confidentiality and privacy, 93b
 contraception, 84
 cultural and diversity awareness, 89–90
 cultural and diversity needs, 64
 differential diagnosis, sexual health and, 77
 ethical dilemmas, 92–94
 ethical training and oversight, 93b
 fertility concerns, female, 65, 70–71, 84–85
 fertility concerns, male, 70–71, 85
 gaps in care, 66
 guidance, offering patients anticipatory and ongoing, 78
 gynecologic care, 79
 legal responsibilities, 91–92
 patient expectations, managing, 94
 presenting problems, 68–72
 presenting problems, and fertility concerns, 72b
 prevalence of sexual dysfunction among cancer survivors, 64
 professional issues and service implementation, 90–95
 psychoeducation, 79–80
 psychosexual maturation, disruption of, 65
 psychosocial issues, 71–72
 psychosocial support, 83–84, 87–88
 reproductive health, 70b, 70–72, 84–89
 reproductive health, assessment of, 74–76, 76t
 reproductive health, care in survivorship, 88–89
 reproductive health, decision support, 87
 reproductive health, resources, 86–87
 risk-taking behaviors, 65
 safer sex practices, 84
 sex and intimacy, broadening definitions of, 78–79, 82–83
 sexual health, assessment of, 73–74
 sexual health, clinical management for females, 80–81
 sexual health, clinical management for males, 82
 sexual health, clinical management of, 77–80
 sexual health, questions to guide discussions, 67t
 sexual intimacy, challenges presented by, 69–70
 sexuality, normalizing discussion of, 78
 sexual problems frequently encountered, 68b
 social support, 70
anxiety and depression, among LGBT patients, 48
antidepressant side-effects, 125
arousal
 and Basson's model of sexual response, 102f
 presenting problems in arousal phase, 101, 101f

behaviors, risk-taking among adolescents and young adults, 65
bereavement care, couples and, 152–55
BETTER Model, of sexual health information, 26b, 36–37
biomedical interventions, psychosexual therapy and, 131–33

Index

biopsychosocial clinical management, and psychosexual therapy, 133–35
biopsychosocial formulation, and assessment, 126
bladder cancer, 118t
body image, in adolescents and young adults, 68–69
bras, 114
breast cancer
  and Female Sexual Function Index, 73
  resources for patients, 111, 114
  sexual consequences of treatment, 99t, 109, 115, 118t, 122
  and sexual needs of gender- and sexuality-diverse women, 56
  sexuality-related communication for women with, 26b
breasts, potential impacts of surgery, 22t

cancer, prevalence of, 1
cancer care, couples and
  advanced cancer, approaches to, 152–55
  anger challenges, 144
  assessment, potential confounding challenges, 147
  assessment principles, 145–48
  background, 139–42
  bereavement care, 152–55
  boundary challenges, 144
  care teams and supervision, 156
  case study, 147–48
  clinical management, 148–50, 149f
  communication issues, 143–44, 151–52
  conflict challenges, 144
  conjoint sessions, reasons to consider, 142
  couple-based therapies, efficacy of, 141
  death and dying, discussing, 152, 153
  differential diagnosis, 148
  emotion-focused therapy, 152–53
  ethical dilemmas, 156
  examining cancer-related impact, 150
  intimacy, revising definitions of, 150–51
  intimacy challenges, 144–45
  intimacy-enhancing couple therapy, 153–54
  key predicaments in couple presentations, 145
  legal responsibilities, 155
  meaning-centered couple therapy, 154–55
  normalizing feelings, 150–51
  policies regarding, 155
  professional issues and service implementation, 155–56
  relationship factors and adjustment to cancer, 140–42
  risk factors for separation or divorce, 139–40
  role challenges, 142–43
  staff records and communications, 155
  supportive processes, identifying, 152
  transition challenges, 143
cancer treatment, impact on sexual functioning and well-being, 21–23, 99t
  chemotherapy, 22–23
  emotional consequences of changes, 23
  frequently reported problems, 116
  hormone therapy, 23, 122
  pelvic surgery, 21, 25b, 71, 122
  prevalence of sexual problems, 115
  radiation therapy, 21–22, 71, 122
  relationship consequences of changes, 23–24, 116
care gaps, for adolescents and young adults, 66
cervical cancer, effects, 118t
chemotherapy, impact on sexual functioning and well-being, 22–23
clinicians
  views on fertility-preservation procedures, 7–8
clitoris,
  and impacts of pelvic surgery on sexuality, 22t
  and sexual pleasure aids, 131–33, 132t
clitoral pumps, 132t
cognitive-behavioral therapy, and adolescents and young adults, 83
colorectal cancer, effects, 118t
communication issues
  couples and cancer care, 143–44, 151–52
  LGBT patient and provider interactions, 47
  strengthening communication skills, 151–52
communication issues, in provision of sexual health support, 30
  barriers to communication, 25b, 26b, 30–33
  barriers to communication, overcoming, 35–36
  cancer patients and their partners, 26b, 36–37, 143–44
  healthcare-professional perspective on, 25b, 26b, 30–31
  patient perspective on, 26b, 31–33

Index

confidentiality and privacy, with adolescents and young adults, 93b
contraception, and psychosocial support of adolescents and young adults, 84
counseling
  in onco-fertility support provision, 12–14
  psychological interventions, 14, 29
  in psychosexual therapy, 127–30
  timing in onco-fertility support, 3–4
couples, and cancer care
  advanced cancer, approaches to, 152–55
  anger challenges, 144
  assessment, potential confounding challenges, 147
  assessment principles, 145–48
  background, 139–42
  bereavement care, 152–55
  boundary challenges, 144
  care teams and supervision, 156
  case study, 147–48
  clinical management, 148–50, 149f
  communication issues, 143–44, 151–52
  conflict challenges, 144
  conjoint sessions, reasons to consider, 142
  couple-based therapies, efficacy of, 141
  couple therapy, 150–52
  death and dying, discussing, 152, 153
  differential diagnosis, 148
  emotion-focused therapy, 152–53
  ethical dilemmas, 156
  examining cancer-related impact, 150
  intimacy, revising definitions of, 150–51
  intimacy challenges, 144–45

intimacy-enhancing couple therapy, 153–54
key predicaments in couple presentations, 145
legal responsibilities, 155
meaning-centered couple therapy, 154–55
normalizing feelings, 150–51
policies regarding, 155
professional issues and service implementation, 155–56
relationship factors and adjustment to cancer, 140–42
risk factors for separation or divorce, 139–40
role challenges, 142–43
staff records and communications, 155
supportive processes, identifying, 152
transition challenges, 143
cultural and diversity awareness, with adolescents and young adults, 89–90
cultural competency training, and serving LGBT patients, 59
cultural issues, young adults and adolescents
  age and maturity, ethical dilemmas, 92–94
  assessment, 72–76
  background of, 63–68
  body image, 68–69, 74
  cancer treatment, indirect effects on sexual health, 69b
  care team communication and records, 90–91
  care team policy, training, and supervision, 94–95
  childhood cancer survivors, 64–65
  clinical management, 77–89
  clinical practice guidelines, 66–68

cognitive-behavioral therapy, 83
confidentiality and privacy, 93b
contraception, 84
cultural and diversity awareness, 89–90
cultural and diversity needs, 64
differential diagnosis, sexual health and, 77
ethical dilemmas, 92–94
ethical training and oversight, 93b
fertility concerns, female, 65, 70–71, 84–85
fertility concerns, male, 70–71, 85
gaps in care, 66
guidance, offering patients anticipatory and ongoing, 78
gynecologic care, 79
legal responsibilities, 91–92
patient expectations, managing, 94
presenting problems, 68–72
presenting problems, and fertility concerns, 72b
prevalence of sexual dysfunction among cancer survivors, 64
professional issues and service implementation, 90–95
psychoeducation, 79–80
psychosexual maturation, disruption of, 65
psychosocial issues, 71–72
psychosocial support, 83–84, 87–88
reproductive health, 70b, 70–72, 84–89
reproductive health, assessment of, 74–76, 76t
reproductive health, care in survivorship, 88–89
reproductive health, decision support, 87
reproductive health, resources, 86–87
risk-taking behaviors, 65

Index

cultural issues, young adults and adolescents (*cont.*)
- sex and intimacy, broadening definitions of, 78–79, 82–83
- sexual health, assessment of, 73–74
- sexual health, clinical management for females, 80–81
- sexual health, clinical management for males, 82
- sexual health, clinical management of, 77–80
- sexual health, questions to guide discussions, 67t
- sexual intimacy, challenges presented by, 69–70
- sexuality, normalizing discussion of, 78
- sexual problems frequently encountered, 68b
- social support, 70

dating
- adolescents and young adults, 64, 65, 69b, 71
- and LGBTQI adolescents and young adults, 90

death and dying, discussing in couple therapy, 152, 153

depression, *vs.* grief, 125–26

depression and anxiety, among LGBT patients, 48

desire, sexual
- and cancer treatment in men, 20
- and chemotherapy in women, 22–23
- and hormone therapy for cancer, 23
- and hormone therapy for hypoactive sexual desire, 107t
- among intimacy challenges, 144–45
- and presenting problems in sexual health, 5, 68b
- screening for decreased, 73

dilators, vaginal, 81
- as biomedical intervention, 25b, 127, 131–33
- and sex after cancer treatment, 25b

dyspareunia
- and effects of cancer treatment, 118t
- and hormone therapy, 23
- and human sexual response cycle, 101f
- and impacts of pelvic surgery, 22t
- presenting problems in sexual health, 68b
- and radiation therapy in women, 22
- sexual difficulties, precipitating and maintaining, 99t
- vaginal dilators to treat, 81

ejaculation
- premature ejaculation, resources for care 114
- retrograde ejaculation, 101

emotion-focused therapy, couples and, 152–53

erectile dysfunction
- among adolescents and young adults, 69, 82
- case study, 109, 123–24
- and cognitive-behavioral therapy, 83
- gay men and concerns regarding, 57
- and low testosterone, 123
- after prostate cancer, 20, 26b
- after radiation treatment, 22
- referral to treatment, 25b
- and sexual consequences of cancer treatment, 99t
- stepped approach to treatment of, 105
- treatment for, 106, 107t

estradiol treatment, 132t

ethics, common dilemmas, 93b
- with adolescents and young adults, 92–94
- in couple therapy, 156
- in onco-fertility support, 14–15
- in psychosexual and psychoeducational issues, 110
- in sexual health support, 37–38

existentially oriented therapy, couples and, 152–53

family building survivorship continuum and care, 5–6

fertility
- evaluation before and after treatment, 9–10
- fertility, effects of oncologic treatment on, 2
- gonadotoxic risk, categories of, 2
- treatments to address, 2

fertility, sexual health and, 3
- unmet needs regarding, 5

fertility concerns, among adolescents and young adults, 65–66, 70–71, 84–85
- presentation of, 72b
- reproductive health, 70b, 70–72

fertility issues
- assessment of, 8–10
- discussing with LGBT patients, 58–59
- discussing with patients, 4–5
- evaluation before and after treatment, 9–10

fertility preservation
- deciding on measures, 3
- indications for counseling on, 8–9
- information and counseling, provision of, 12–14
- in men, 12
- in women, 10–11
- in women, case study, 12

fertility preservation procedures

barriers and
facilitators, 6–8
Flibanserin, 131–33
foreplay
and expanded sexual
repertoire, 131
and sexual pleasure
aids, 132t

gonadotoxic risk,
categories of, 2
grief
naming and
normalizing, 152
vs. depression, 125–26
gynecologic care,
importance for
adolescents and young
adults, 79

head and neck cancer,
effects of treatment,
115–16, 118t
healthcare professionals
views on fertility-
preservation
procedures, 7–8
hormone replacement
therapy, 70b,
105, 123
hormone therapy, impact
on sexual functioning
and well-being,
23, 122
human immunodeficiency
virus (HIV), stigma
and cancers associated
with, 48–49
human papillomavirus
(HPV), stigma and
cancers associated
with, 48–49
human sexual response
cycle, phases of, 101f,
101–2, 102f

impotence. See erectile
dysfunction
incontinence, 118t
and avoiding sex, 54, 57
and climacturia, 101
after radiation
treatment, 21–22
supportive counseling
for, 129–30
after surgery, 21

and treatment for
prostate cancer,
20, 22t
intimacy-enhancing couple
therapy, 153–54

law
legal implications
of onco-fertility
support, 15
legal responsibilities,
couples and cancer
care, 155
legal responsibilities,
psychosexual and
psychoeducational
issues, 110
legal responsibilities, with
adolescents and young
adults, 91–92
lesbian, gay, bisexual,
and transgender
(LGBT) patient-care
issues
antidiscrimination
policies, instituting, 60
background of, 41–45
barriers to quality cancer
care, 45
cancer care, and
knowledge
gaps, 44–45
cancer care, experience
of, 42b, 44
cancer care, issues
complicating, 42b
cancer population, 43
case study, 52, 56, 58
cisgender and
heterosexual identities,
assuming in patients,
46, 50, 52
clinical management,
recommendations
for, 42b, 49–54
cultural competency
training for
staff, 59
definitions and scope,
41–43, 42b
depression and
anxiety, 48
disclosure of SOGI,
facilitating, 50–75
fertility issues,
discussing, 58–59

gay and bisexual men,
providing support
for, 56–58
gender- and sexuality-
diverse women,
providing support
for, 56
healthcare
environment, 49
heteronormativity, 46
human immunodeficiency
virus (HIV), stigma
and cancers associated
with, 48–49
human papillomavirus
(HPV), stigma and
cancers associated
with, 48–49
knowledge gaps, cancer
care and, 44–45
LGBT advocacy,
facilitating, 60
LGBT rights, 43–44
minority stress
theory, 43
nontraditional
relationships
and support
networks, 47–48
partners and families of
choice, 51–54
patient-centered care,
providing, 51
patient-provider
interactions, 47
professional issues
and service
implementation, 59–61
resources and support
groups, identifying,
42b, 52
resources and support
groups, increasing
access to, 61
resources and
support groups,
lack of, 47
sexual health, providing
support for,
42b, 54–58
sexual orientation
and gender
identity, disclosure
of, 47, 60
stigma and
discrimination, 45, 48

Index

libido
  among adolescents and young adults, 68, 71, 81, 82
  in biopsychosocial formulation, 126
  after cancer treatment, 116, 122–23
  and chemotherapy, 22–23
  in couples, 151, 153
  encouraging sex despite reduced, 111

massage, and intimacy after cancer, 25b, 82–83, 89
mastectomy
  cultural significance of, 118t
  potential impacts of, 22t
  and sexual orientation/gender identity, 51
meaning-centered couple therapy, 154–55
men, fertility preservation in, 12
mindfulness meditation, as psychosocial intervention, 130
minority stress theory, and LGBT issues, 43

onco-fertility support, provision of
  assessment of fertility issues, 8–10
  background, 1–5
  cancer prevalence, 1
  clinical management, 10–12
  counseling and information, 12–14
  ethical dilemmas, 14–15
  evaluation of fertility before and after treatment, 9–10
  family building, survivorship continuum and care, 5–6
  fertility and sexual health, 3, 5
  fertility issues, discussing with patients, 4–5
  fertility preservation, case study, 12
  fertility preservation, deciding on measures, 3
  fertility preservation, indications for counseling on, 8–9
  fertility preservation, in men, 12
  fertility preservation, in women, 10–11
  fertility preservation procedures, barriers and facilitators, 6–8
  gonadotoxic risk, categories of, 2
  legal implications, 15
  onco-fertility, as emerging discipline, 2
  onco-fertility, definition of, 2
  oncologic treatment, effects on fertility, 2
  presenting problems, 5–8
  professional issues, 12–15
  psychological interventions, 14
  service implementation, 12–15
  timing of counseling, 3–4
orgasm, 101
  brain surgery, impact of, 99t
  and models of sexual response, 101–2, 101f
  pain with, 124, 133

pain
  during intercourse, 124
  during intercourse, case study, 109
  during orgasm, 101, 133
  postcoital, 101f
  psychoeducation regarding, 79
papaverin injection, 132t
partners, and risk of not receiving sexual health information, 34
patient-centered care, providing to LGBT patients, 51
patients
  communication issues, perspective on, 26b, 31–33
  discussing fertility issues with, 4–5
  discussing sexual dysfunction with, 102–3
  family building, survivorship continuum and care, 5–6
  guide to sexual aids for, 132t
  patient expectations, managing, 94
  providing information and counseling to, 12–14
  psychological interventions for, 14, 29
  views on fertility-preservation procedures, 6–7
patients, provision of sexual health information to cancer patients and their partners, 26b, 36–37
  culturally and linguistically diverse patients, 35
  LGBTQI patients, 35
  older patients, 34–35
  See also lesbian, gay, bisexual, and transgender (LGBT) patient-care issues
pelvic surgery, impact on sexuality, 21, 25b, 71, 122
penis
  intracavernosal injection, 82
  length loss, treatment for, 107t
penectomy, 22t
penile prosthesis, 132t
prostatectomy, effects of, 57
petting, and normalizing affection and intimacy, 153
peyronie curvature of penis, 132t
phosphodiesterase type 5 inhibitor, 107t, 131, 132t
  avanafil, 132t
  sildenafil, 132t

tadalafil, 132*t*
vardenafil, 132*t*
PLISSIT Model, of sexual health information, 24–28, 25*f*
  intensive therapy, 25*b*, 27–28
  limited information, providing, 24–26, 25*b*
  permission to discuss sex, 24, 25*b*
  specific suggestions, offering, 25*b*, 26–27
privacy and confidentiality, with adolescents and young adults, 93*b*
prostaglandin E injection, tablet, 132*t*
prostate cancer, effects, 118*t*
prostatectomy, 22*t*
  and sexual behavior of gay and bisexual men, 57
  sexual consequences of, 99*t*
psychoeducation, for adolescents and young adults, 79–80
psychoeducational issues, interventions for
  background of, 98–100
  biomedical interventions, 105
  care teams and supervision, 111
  clinical management, 104–9
  clinical management, of erectile dysfunction, 109
  clinical management, of painful intercourse, 109
  differential diagnosis, investigations for, 103–4
  ethical dilemmas, 110
  human sexual response cycle, phases of, 101*f*, 101–2, 102*f*
  legal responsibilities, 110
  men, clinical management of key issues for, 107*t*, 109

patient records and staff communications, 110
patient-reported outcome measures, 103–4
policies, 110
presenting problems, 101–3
professional issues and service implementation, 110–12
psychosocial interventions, 105–7
safe sex and other considerations, 108–9
sexual difficulties, factors for, 104*b*
sexual dysfunction, discussing with patients, 102–3
sexual dysfunction, stepped approach to clinical management, 105
sexual rehabilitation, approaches to, 108*f*
sexual rehabilitation, for individuals and couples, 111–12
training modules, 111
women, clinical management of key issues for, 106*t*, 109
psychological interventions, provision of, 14, 29
psychosexual issues, interventions for
  background of, 98–100
  biomedical interventions, 105
  care teams and supervision, 111
  clinical management, 104–9
  clinical management, of erectile dysfunction, 109
  clinical management, of painful intercourse, 109
  differential diagnosis, investigations for, 103–4
  ethical dilemmas, 110

human sexual response cycle, phases of, 101*f*, 101–2, 102*f*
legal responsibilities, 110
men, clinical management of key issues for, 107*t*, 109
patient records and staff communications, 110
patient-reported outcome measures, 103–4
policies, 110
presenting problems, 101–3
professional issues and service implementation, 110–12
psychosocial interventions, 105–7
safe sex and other considerations, 108–9
sexual difficulties, factors for, 104*b*
sexual dysfunction, discussing with patients, 102–3
sexual dysfunction, stepped approach to clinical management, 105
sexual rehabilitation, approaches to, 108*f*
sexual rehabilitation, for individuals and couples, 111–12
training modules, 111
women, clinical management of key issues for, 106*t*, 109
psychosexual maturation, disruptions in adolescents and young adults, 65
psychosexual therapy, relationships and access to
  expertise, 135–37
  background, 115–17
  biomedical interventions, 131–33
  biopsychosocial formulation, 126
  cancer treatment, impact on relationships, 116

Index

psychosexual therapy, relationships and (cont.)
- clinical management, 127–35, 128f
- clinical management, biopsychosocial, 133–35
- comorbidities, 125b, 125–26
- confounding issues, 123
- couples sex therapy, 131, 132t
- couples sex therapy, case study, 134–35
- depression vs. grief, 125–26
- differential diagnosis, investigations for, 124–26
- differential diagnosis, key differentials, 124–25
- differential diagnosis and, 124–25
- expanding sexual repertoire, 131
- frequently reported sexual problems, 116
- individual sex therapy, 130, 132t
- mindfulness meditation, 130
- presenting problems, case study, 123–24
- presenting problems, key symptoms and signs, 117–23
- professional issues and service implementation, 135–37
- psychosocial interventions, 127–31, 129t
- sensate focus exercises, 130–31
- sexual aids for patients, guide to, 132t
- sexual communication, special considerations, 117b
- sexual dysfunction, defining, 116
- sexual function, assessment of, 124
- sexual problems, by cancer type, 118t
- supportive counseling, 127–30
- *See also* couples, and cancer care

psychosocial concerns, among adolescents and young adults, 71–72

psychosocial interventions, sexual recovery and, 127–31, 129t

radiation therapy, impact on sexual functioning and well-being, 21–22, 71, 122

relationships, psychosexual therapy and
- access to expertise, 135–37
- assessment, biopsychosocial formulation, 126
- assessment, comorbidities, 125b, 125–26
- assessment, differential diagnosis and, 124–25
- background, 115–17
- biomedical interventions, 131–33
- cancer treatment, impact on relationships, 116
- clinical management, 127–35, 128f
- clinical management, biopsychosocial, 133–35
- confounding issues, in diagnosis and treatment, 123
- couples sex therapy, 131, 132t
- couples sex therapy, case study, 134–35
- depression vs. grief, 125–26
- differential diagnosis, investigations for, 124–26
- differential diagnosis, key differentials, 124–25
- expanding sexual repertoire, 131
- frequently reported sexual problems, 116
- individual sex therapy, 130, 132t
- mindfulness meditation, 130
- presenting problems, case study, 123–24
- presenting problems, key symptoms and signs, 117–23
- professional issues and service implementation, 135–37
- psychosocial interventions, 127–31, 129t
- sensate focus exercises, 130–31
- sexual aids for patients, guide to, 132t
- sexual communication, special considerations, 117b
- sexual dysfunction, defining, 116
- sexual function, assessment of, 124
- sexual problems, by cancer type, 118t
- supportive counseling, 127–30
- *See also* couples, and cancer care

reproductive health, among adolescents and young adults, 70b, 70–72, 84–89
- assessment of, 74–76, 76t

sensate focus exercises, as psychosocial intervention, 130–31

sex therapy
- couples, 131, 132t
- couples, case study, 134–35
- individuals, 130, 132t

sex toys, and sexual rehabilitation, 29, 108f

sexual desire
- and cancer treatment in men, 20
- and chemotherapy in women, 22–23
- and hormone therapy for cancer, 23

and hormone therapy for hypoactive, 107t
among intimacy challenges, 144–45
and presenting problems in sexual health, 5, 68b
screening for decreased, 73
sexual dysfunction, defining, 116
sexual health, among adolescents and young adults assessment of, 73–74
cancer treatment, indirect effects of, 69b
contraception, 84
presenting problems, 68–72
questions to guide discussions, 67t
reproductive health, 70–72
safer sex practices, 84
sexual intimacy, challenges presented by, 69–70
sexual health, fertility and, 3
unmet needs regarding, 5
sexual health, provision of support, 39
access to expertise, 135–37
background, 19–21
to cancer patients and their partners, 26b, 36–37
cancer treatment, impact on sexual function and well-being, 21–23
clinical management, 24–30
clinical management, case study, 29–30
clinical-team training and supervision, 39
communication, barriers to, 25b, 26b, 30–33
communication, healthcare-professional perspective on, 25b, 26b, 30–31
communication, overcoming barriers to, 35–36

communication, patient perspective on, 26b, 31–33
communication issues, 30
effectiveness of support, 29
ethical dilemmas, 37–38
groups at risk of not receiving, 34–35
information and advice, BETTER model, 26b, 36–37
information and advice, PLISSIT Model, 24–28, 25b, 25f
to LGBTQI patients, 35
to older patients, 34–35
policies regarding, 38
presenting problems, 21–24
professional issues and service implementation, 30–39
sexual changes, emotional consequences of, 23
sexual changes, relationship consequences of, 23–24
to sexual partners, 34
sexual identity, terms associated with, 41–43, 42b
sexual intimacy broadening definition of, 78–79, 82–83
couples and cancer care, 144–45
intimacy-enhancing couple therapy, 153–54
revising definitions of, 150–51
sexually transmitted viruses, stigma and, 48–49
sexual orientation and gender identity (SOGI), and patient care See lesbian, gay, bisexual, and transgender (LGBT) patient-care issues
sexual partners, and risk of not receiving sexual health information, 34

sexual problems
by cancer type, 118t
prevalence after cancer treatment, 115
sexual rehabilitation
approaches to, 108f
couples sex therapy, 131, 132t
couples sex therapy, case study, 134–35
expanding sexual repertoire, 131
for individuals and couples, 111–12
individual sex therapy, 130, 132t
mindfulness meditation, 130
psychosocial interventions, 127–31, 129t
sensate focus exercises, 130–31
sexual aids for patients, guide to, 132t
social support, and sexual health among adolescents and young adults, 70
stoma, implications for intimacy and body image, 21, 68–69
substance use, 125, 126
surgery, impact on sexual functioning and well-being, 21, 25b, 71, 122

testicular surgery
and fertility preservation, 12
and gender-confirming procedures, 59
sexual health and, 68, 118t

urinary leakage, as presenting problem, 122

vagina
arousal phase of human sexual response cycle, 101
and cervical cancer, treatment for, 118t

vagina (*cont.*)
  radiation therapy, effects of, 22
  sexual pleasure aids, 132*t*
  vaginal prosthesis, 105
vaginal dilators, 81
  as biomedical intervention, 25*b*, 127, 131–33
  and sex after cancer treatment, 25*b*
viruses, stigma and sexually transmitted, 48–49, 118*t*

women, fertility preservation in, 10–11
  case study, 12

xerostomia, kissing and, 118*t*

young adults, and adolescents
  age and maturity, ethical dilemmas, 92–94
  assessment, 72–76
  background of, 63–68
  body image, 68–69, 74
  cancer treatment, indirect effects on sexual health, 69*b*
  care team communication and records, 90–91
  care team policy, training, and supervision, 94–95
  childhood cancer survivors, 64–65
  clinical management, 77–89
  clinical practice guidelines, 66–68
  cognitive-behavioral therapy, 83
  confidentiality and privacy, 93*b*
  contraception, 84
  cultural and diversity awareness, 89–90
  cultural and diversity needs, 64
  differential diagnosis, sexual health and, 77
  ethical dilemmas, 92–94
  ethical training and oversight, 93*b*
  fertility concerns, female, 65, 70–71, 84–85
  fertility concerns, male, 70–71, 85
  gaps in care, 66
  guidance, offering patients anticipatory and ongoing, 78
  gynecologic care, 79
  legal responsibilities, 91–92
  patient expectations, managing, 94
  presenting problems, 68–72
  presenting problems, and fertility concerns, 72*b*
  prevalence of sexual dysfunction among cancer survivors, 64
  professional issues and service implementation, 90–95
  psychoeducation, 79–80
  psychosexual maturation, disruption of, 65
  psychosocial issues, 71–72
  psychosocial support, 83–84, 87–88
  reproductive health, 70*b*, 70–72, 84–89
  reproductive health, assessment of, 74–76, 76*t*
  reproductive health, care in survivorship, 88–89
  reproductive health, decision support, 87
  reproductive health, resources, 86–87
  risk-taking behaviors, 65
  safer sex practices, 84
  sex and intimacy, broadening definitions of, 78–79, 82–83
  sexual health, assessment of, 73–74
  sexual health, clinical management for females, 80–81
  sexual health, clinical management for males, 82
  sexual health, clinical management of, 77–80
  sexual health, questions to guide discussions, 67*t*
  sexual intimacy, challenges presented by, 69–70
  sexuality, normalizing discussion of, 78
  sexual problems frequently encountered, 68*b*
  social support, 70

www.ingramcontent.com/pod-product-compliance
Ingram Content Group UK Ltd.
Pitfield, Milton Keynes, MK11 3LW, UK
UKHW021258180426
11947UKWH00015B/904